My Voice,
My Choice

My Voice, My Choice

A Practical Guide to Writing a
Meaningful
Healthcare Directive

WHAT MUST BE INCLUDED

WHY THIS MATTERS

TOOLS TO HELP YOU

Anne Elizabeth Denny

Directives by Design, LLC, Minneapolis

Published by:
Directives by Design, LLC
4666 Stonecliffe Drive
Eagan, Minnesota 55122
PlanWellFinishWell.com

Cover design by Amy Kirkpatrick, kirkpatrickdesign.com
Book design by Dorie McClelland, springbookdesign.com
Editing, encouragement, and wonderful suggestions by Connie Anderson

ISBN: 978-0-9859822-0-1 (print)
ISBN: 978-0-9859822-1-8 (ebook)

Contents

HOW

From "Carol's Song" written for my mother,
Carol Easley Denny.

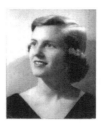

Carol Easley Denny
1934–2012

Through vacant, hollow eyes,
I wonder if you see me.
Am I trapped inside the memories
That your fragile mind erased?
A flickering, fleeting smile,
Brings back your face, reminds me
Of the woman who once raised me.
Is her spirit still alive? Is your spirit still alive?
Can your soul speak what your words may not?
Can your heart hear what your mind may not?
Can you feel my presence? I'm here.
I am here with you, beside you.
Can my love sustain, remind you
You will always be my mother?
And, I'll always be your child.

Introduction

Whoever you are and for whatever reason you are reading this book, welcome. Maybe you recognize your own need and responsibility to write a healthcare directive. Perhaps someone has given you a copy of this book with the hopes that it will open the door for conversation about end-of-life decisions. You might be older, but not necessarily. You might be healthy, or you might be facing a difficult diagnosis. Preparing for the end of life applies to any age and every state of health. Whatever the reason for reading this book, it will inspire and empower you to express your end-of-life healthcare preferences in writing and through meaningful conversation with loved ones.

> Many legal terms are used throughout this book. An explanation for the most important terms is offered in chapter 3. Additionally, a glossary and a list of frequently used acronyms are available at the back of the book.

Preparing thoroughly for the end of life requires much more than writing a healthcare directive. Nonetheless, in this book, I have chosen to remain focused on why and how to write a meaningful healthcare directive because I believe this is the best place to start. Each of us deserves to receive all of the healthcare treatment, and only the treatment, that is right for us at the end of our life. A well-written healthcare directive communicates our treatment preferences, should we be unable to do so. It is also important to note that while healthcare directives are most frequently used in end-of-life situations, having your treatment preferences documented and available will be invaluable to those providing your care and making decisions on your behalf if you should ever become temporarily incapacitated due to an accident or a sudden medical event.

Dr. Ira Byock, a practicing physician and head of Palliative Care at the Dartmouth-Hitchcock Medical Center in New England, writes that the dying process is more personal than it is medical. I agree with Dr. Byock. As you read this book, I hope to help you explore your thoughts and emotions so you may prepare yourself and your loved ones for the personal nature of the dying process.

Advances in medical technology have skewed our perspective. Whereas the dying process used to occur naturally at home in the presence of loved ones, the process has morphed into a technology-driven chase to extend life. If a patient's wishes are not known, medical decision-makers will quickly fill the vacuum. Doctors are trained to fight death until the bitter end, if they have no instructions stating otherwise.

> For a comprehensive discussion on all aspects of end-of-life care, I recommend Jane Brody's *Guide to the Great Beyond,* Jo Myers' *Good to Go,* and Dr. Ira Byock's books, *Dying Well* and *Best Care Possible.*

As a society, and as individuals, we have the opportunity to reclaim the personal nature of the dying process. Writing and communicating our end-of-life preferences is where it begins.

My mother lived with Alzheimer's for twenty years. She did not know me for the final eight years of her life. Watching my mother retreat into a shell profoundly impacted my view of living with a meaningful quality of life. My family experience makes me an unwilling expert about the journey towards the end of life. I am a champion from the most personal level.

I am not an attorney, nor a physician, thus I do not provide any legal or medical advice. What I have learned about end-of-life matters comes from a great deal of research, talking to families, attorneys, and doctors—and from my own family experience. I want to use my experience and that of many individuals whom I have interviewed, to help you learn to be open with your family about your healthcare treatment wishes. I have a heartfelt desire to ease the burden of end-of-life decisions for loved ones, as well as helping individuals to approach the end of life with less fear, anxiety, and uncertainty.

In addition to writing this book, I have designed and developed a website that helps individuals write a meaningful healthcare directive. I invite you to visit the site at www.PlanWellFinishWell.com to learn more.

My Voice, My Choice is a practical guide, written as a handbook. It addresses **why** healthcare directives matter, **what** should be included in a well-written document, and **how** to go about creating yours. It strives to educate you, prepare you, motivate you, and empower you to write a meaningful healthcare directive.

I would like to acknowledge and thank Oakwood Healthcare in Dearborn, Michigan, for allowing me to use the phrase *My Voice, My Choice*—for which Oakwood owns the trademark—as my title. The Oakwood system offers an advance healthcare directive tool free of charge for the individuals and communities it serves. The tool can be found at: www.oakwood.org/advance-directives.

Because end-of-life planning involves numerous terms and several types of documents, *My Voice, My Choice* includes some repetition that I believe is warranted because it will strengthen your understanding of healthcare directives. This repetition is intentional and was done with clarity for the reader in mind. Additionally, I am using **his** and **her** interchangeably for ease of reading.

This book presents two challenges. First, let your voice be heard now—make your end-of-life choices known. It's much easier when no health crisis is looming, no one is in tears, or no one has lost mental clarity. Be a catalyst for your family by writing and sharing your healthcare directive. Secondly, embrace the opportunity to inspire others. Add a personal note, and give this book to loved ones to help open the door for end-of-life discussion.

Let's start the conversation *now*.

WHY

Why should I invest the time to write a healthcare directive?

Do it for yourself.

Ensure that your end-of-life healthcare preferences are clearly understood and followed.

**Do it for those you love,
and who love you.**

Give your loved ones peace of mind by empowering them to honor your end-of-life wishes.

1

Bad Death or Good Death: Which Will Yours Be?

Everyone knows someone who has died. You do and I do. Everyone has a story. Some stories might be recent, some from long ago. Some stories remind you of a close loved one or a dear friend. Others offer a vague recollection of an elderly relative or a business colleague.

One hundred years ago, most stories about the passing of a loved one looked about the same. Family members cared for the sick and dying at home. Family gathered around a loved one, comforting one another as they watched life wane from a father, mother, brother, sister, grandparent, or child. The signs of impending death were recognized and accepted. Death was familiar to most and was woven into the fabric of family life.

Fast forward to the last few decades. Technological advances have propelled us into an era where death is medically managed, not family-managed. The line between prolonging the dying process, versus extending life, has become difficult to identify. Dr. Jeff Gordon, of Grant Medical Center in Ohio, states: "Today's high-tech medical care can sustain technical life—the beating heart—but utterly fails to restore real quality of life for many. There comes a point when physicians can prolong dying, but not provide quality living."[1] In general, society pushes the line, often unreasonably, with technology-driven care. Yet each case is individual, affecting a circle of loved ones. The ability to extend life through machines and medication has created emotional, ethical, and spiritual dilemmas for many families such as:

- When do we say, "Enough!" to the healthcare professional offering another treatment, another surgery, or another medication to a dying loved one?

- How can we know when it is time to allow death to occur or when to zealously pursue all possible treatment?

- How do we know when it is time to pull the plug?

- How can families remain united in comforting their loved one and each other?

A Bad Death

As Baby Boomers age, more and more families will struggle through the difficult death of a loved one. Sadly, many tragic stories will ensue. Ill-prepared children will see their parent's declining health as a problem to fix, instead of a natural process to honor. They will overlook signs that the dying process has begun.

As Dr. Ira Byock states in his book, *Dying Well*,[2] what many families don't realize is there can be something worse than watching a loved one die—watching a loved one die badly. One of the unintended consequences of our advanced technology is the reality that the dying process, when prolonged, can cause needless suffering.

A bad death has one or more of the following characteristics:

- The patient receives *undesired* medical care. Typically, this includes interventions such as C.P.R. (cardiopulmonary resuscitation), intubation (ventilation), or other heroic measures that the patient, if able to speak for himself, may not have chosen.

8

- Often the patient endures a long, slow decline in Intensive Care, hooked up to machines and/or tied with restraints to prevent her from pulling out tubes, and she never recovers.

- Loved ones must ultimately choose to pull the plug.

- The patient experiences unnecessary suffering.

- Loved ones square off in bitter disagreement over treatment decisions for the patient. Lawsuits can result. Families become divided when they most need to be united in support for the dying patient and for one another.

A bad death represents a futile battle against the inevitability of death. Decisions in a crisis can be driven by hope, fear, and a complex mix of emotions. The human instinct for survival is strong, so we viscerally fight against death. We might have unfinished emotional business, so we consent to treatment, hoping for more time to resolve issues and make peace.

Aggressive and excessive treatment can cause unintended consequences, resulting in heartbreak for families and suffering for the patient. Imagine the anguish for the patient's loved ones when resuscitation restores a heart rhythm, only to have them realize the person's brain function has been so profoundly compromised that she remains in a persistent vegetative state.

Absent the patient's voice through written instructions, decision-makers feel compelled to authorize all possible care and hope for the best. The courage to withhold or withdraw treatment could spare suffering and allow a good death. Yet, by authorizing all possible care we dodge the possibility of guilty feelings or the perceived judgment of others.

Paul's story portrays what families face every day in society. He shares the story of how his father passed away in 2008, just two short years after his mother passed away.

> While I lived in town close to my father, my brother John lived on the East Coast, and came to visit only every few years. John had not visited since Mom died and did not come when Dad's health took a turn for the worse.
>
> One evening, Dad began to experience difficulty breathing. An ambulance took him to the hospital where the doctors diagnosed end-stage lung cancer. What a surprise, since Dad never smoked. The doctors thought he might only have two months to live. Though I realized Dad's health had been declining, I hadn't wanted to talk about his death after Mom died. I didn't want to alarm him, and I was in denial.
>
> Dad's condition worsened. When I finally grasped the reality of Dad's decline, I asked Dad his wishes. He said he didn't want to be kept alive on machines; he said he wanted a natural death. Unfortunately, he never shared his wishes with John. Nor did he ever record his choices legally. Since neither my brother nor I was listed as health-care agent, neither one of us had final authority. I felt I should be the decision-maker since I lived close to Dad, and we had at least talked about his wishes. My brother disagreed vehemently. As the older son, John felt he should be in charge.

My brother flew into town when the end was near. He wanted everything possible done to keep Dad alive. I advocated allowing Dad to die a natural death, but my brother pushed for aggressive treatment. I think he felt guilty for all the times he had not come to visit. I could see John wishing for more time with Dad to resolve their differences and the unfinished business between them.

I watched Dad waste away in Intensive Care for six weeks. He was on a ventilator, had no control over his own bodily functions, had a feeding tube, became emaciated, and even developed a bedsore. For the last two weeks, he was in and out of consciousness and barely spoke to us. In the last few days, he didn't even seem to recognize us or know we were present. It was absolutely horrible.

If Dad had written down his wishes and had designated me as his healthcare agent, he could have had a peaceful, dignified passing. Instead it was torture for him and for us. I would have said no to a ventilator, to C.P.R., and to the feeding tube. Instead, the doctors, though trying to do their best, broke a rib giving him C.P.R. Dad's hands were tied to the bed rail to prevent him from pulling out his feeding tube. Unfortunately, his feeding tube caused an infection.

I'm still so angry at John, I haven't spoken to him since Dad's funeral, and that was three years ago.

Countless families have experienced a similar tragedy. Watching a loved one die badly compounds the grief of loss.

Reclaiming the Dying Process

Control of the dying process needs to return to the patient and the family. All that medical science has to offer can still be leveraged, albeit wisely, appropriately, and within the patient's preferences. In their book, *OK to Die,*[3] authors Dr. Monica Williams-Murphy and Kristian Murphy suggest we need to shift from "high-tech to high-touch medicine" at the end of life.

The birthing process offers an example of a medical practice and life stage that has evolved to a patient-centered experience. Before the mid-'80s, the birthing process belonged to the doctor and the hospital. The expectant mother was rolled into a surgical suite and put under sedation. The father anxiously paced the hallway. The baby was delivered and moved to the infant nursery, while the mom was rolled back to her room to recover. The father would greet his sleepy wife and proclaim, "We have a beautiful baby girl." Grandparents would anxiously await a phone call.

My, how things have changed. Now, expectant parents plan their baby's birth—choosing the hospital birthing suite or in-home delivery; doctor, midwife or doula; natural birth, water birth, pain medication or epidural; music, aromatherapy, video-taping, family present (or not); and countless other possibilities. While parents may script the desired birth process, healthcare professionals and all the available technology stand at the ready to intervene when complications arise. The obstetrician can decide in an instant to perform an emergency C-section. Thorough planning gives parents a sense of control, and in most cases, results in a memorable birthing experience.

Like the birthing process, patients and families can reclaim the highly personal dying process. Experiences for patients and their families during the dying process could be so different if:

• Individuals scripted their own end-of-life preferences.

- Families openly discussed each member's end-of-life plan.

- Physicians became more willing to acknowledge the dying process in order to help families recognize the opportunity to care for their loved one according to a written end-of-life plan.

A Good Death

How would you define a good death? Even if the dying process unfolds over time, a patient can experience a peaceful passing and a good death. A good death has the following qualities:

- Being at peace spiritually,

- Being at peace with, and feeling supported by, loved ones,

- Knowing one's life has had purpose and value,

- Having one's affairs in order,

- Living symptom-free, and pain-free final days,

- Experiencing dignified and gentle final hours without aggressive, invasive treatment,

- Feeling a sense of control by having one's treatment decisions honored, and

- Knowing loved ones are united in their support and love for each other.

While none of us can predict the circumstances of our death, thorough preparations will go a long way to assuring a good death. A well-written healthcare directive that has been communicated to your physician and your family, coupled with a strong healthcare agent advocating on your behalf, addresses many of these characteristics. The emotional and spiritual work of a life well lived addresses the rest.

Susan's story shows how a healthcare directive clearly communicated her wishes to her medical team and to her family.

Susan was a widow. Though she was lonely at times and missed her husband, at sixty-nine years old she was still active physically, quite social, and her mind was razor-sharp. She lived alone and relished her independence.

When Susan turned seventy, she invited her three children out to lunch. She gave each of them a copy of her healthcare directive. She walked them through her preferences, giving everyone a chance to ask questions. The discussion was awkward at times, but Susan was determined to have her wishes followed when her time came.

Susan appointed her younger brother as her primary healthcare agent, so none of the children would feel the weight of making difficult healthcare decisions if any were required. Her pastor had agreed to serve as the alternate agent. She had a private meeting with her brother and pastor to discuss her decisions. She also discussed her preferences with her internist.

Every year thereafter on her birthday, Susan sent a note to her children, her brother, and her pastor to let them know her wishes were still the same. Whenever she met with her doctor, they reviewed her wishes.

At eighty-four years old, Susan suffered a severe stroke. Her daughter found her collapsed by her bed one afternoon. Since Susan was still in her nightgown, her daughter knew the incident had occurred during the night. Susan was transported to the hospital and evaluated in the emergency room. Susan's daughter called her uncle (named as healthcare agent) and her mother's pastor immediately. The emergency room physician spoke to Susan's brother and her doctor by phone and learned Susan's wishes.

Damage to her brain was significant, rendering her unable to speak and also paralyzed on one side. At the request of her brother, Susan's doctor consulted with the hospital. All agreed that in this situation, Susan would not want to pursue curative treatment. Music was played by her bedside, as she had requested. Family and friends were notified, and those that could, visited. Though Susan couldn't speak, she would respond to touch and made every effort to smile or nod. Susan had expressed anxiety about being left alone to die, so her brother, pastor, and children all took turns staying near her side. Susan's medical team managed her symptoms so she did not suffer. A second stroke occurred on the tenth day. Susan died peacefully; her children remained united and able to love and comfort one another. Susan's wishes were honored.

Susan's was a good death. She was in her mid-eighties and had lived a good, mostly healthy life. Because of Susan's proactive communication with her loved ones and her physician, her wishes were known and followed.

Variations on Paul's and Susan's stories are endless. For Paul's father, dying was lengthy and anguishing. The relationship between brothers was deeply damaged. For Susan, the dying process was not disrupted by undesired, aggressive treatment. Her death was as she wished—gentle and dignified. Susan's family remained united in their love and support for her and for each other.

There are good deaths and there are bad, even horrible deaths. Reflect on the stories of those who have passed away. Was theirs a good death?

Saying Goodbye Twice

My family story reflects a different kind of death. They say that with Alzheimer's disease, you grieve twice. You grieve as your loved one slips away. You grieve when they finally let go.

In the summer of 1994, at the age of sixty, my mother was formally diagnosed with Alzheimer's disease. Her mother and several of her aunts and uncles fell victim to this horrible disease. Mom dreaded Alzheimer's and resisted the idea of being labeled. Although the symptoms were evident for some time, our family delayed pursuing Mom's diagnosis. Our hearts were torn between denial and acceptance.

Our family story has been shaped by Mom's journey through Alzheimer's. I watched helplessly as my mom lost her ability to communicate. She did not know who I was for eight long years. I did not hear Mom speak an intelligible word for the final five years of her life. In the last year, her eyes rarely opened and when they did open, all I saw was a glazed, vacant look.

Through all those years, I watched my father care lovingly for my mother. I admired and respected my father's devotion. Caring for a spouse with Alzheimer's disease is an enormous challenge. Many caregivers say it is both a gift and a burden. I observed this in my father's care for my mother. Serving in the role of caregiver softened my father, exposing a more tender heart. Yet the burden of caring for my mom at home compromised his health. Consumed with Mom's care, Dad was essentially cut off from his social support system. He cared for Mom in their home for nine years. During that time, he became sleep-deprived. And his emotional and physical exhaustion were clearly evident. I worried that I would lose both parents as a result of Alzheimer's disease.

For eleven years, my mother lived in a wonderful nursing home with caring, attentive staff. My father visited her almost every day. Knowing that she was well cared for and safe allowed my father to live a full life, engaging in activities and enjoying social connections.

If my parents had discussed the course of her disease when she was still mentally capable, I believe my mother would have advised Dad to move her to a nursing home sooner, rather than later. I think my mother would have been heartbroken to know how the demands of her care affected my father. Thankfully, I believe the Alzheimer's disease rendered her unaware.

In her last few months, Mom slept about twenty hours a day. Her wakefulness was limited to short intervals. She could not eat or drink on her own, or attend to any of her own care or personal hygiene.

> In her final weeks, Mom was bedridden. Swallowing became increasingly difficult. She did not respond to my voice or the touch of my hand. The mother I knew had withdrawn into a shell, and I could not reach her. I knew Mom was dying.
>
> In May of 2012, Mom experienced a sharp decline. Mom's breathing was labored. She stopped eating and drinking. She had a fever, so the nurse practitioner asked if we wanted to order tests to determine the source of infection. We pursued comfort care only. After three long days of watching life wane from her body, her spirit was set free. Mom was finally released from the prison of Alzheimer's disease on May 27th.
>
> I share our family story because it is familiar, and will become familiar, to many. Discussing end-of-life choices while we are healthy and mentally capable is an urgent call to action for every adult.

In Summary

While none of us can know what circumstances will befall us, developing a plan for the dying process gives each of us the ability to define what we *can* control. We can prepare for a good death. Use this book as a guide to help you develop your plan. Writing a comprehensive healthcare directive is the first step of your plan. Communicating your wishes is the second step. The final step is to live life fully in the present, knowing you and your loved ones are prepared for whatever the future brings.

2

Getting Real About Our Mortality

As a society, we've developed a real aversion to death. Some cultures are far more realistic about recognizing death as a part of life. Taking time to think about end-of-life preferences first requires us to face our mortality. It reminds us that our days are numbered. Pondering the end of our life may stir up a flood of emotions as we reflect on our past and recognize our future is finite. Denial seems easier.

A Snapshot of Reality

Why do we all think *that will never happen to me*? Here are a few realities to consider:

1. Chronic disease is the primary cause of death.

Did you know that 70 percent of Americans will die from a chronic disease?[4] Think about the medical implications for the end of life for those with diabetes, obesity, heart disease, respiratory disease, kidney disease, and cancer. Thus for seven out of every ten of us, our health will decline over time. For the majority, dying will be a process, not an event.

2. Few of us will die unexpectedly.

In fact, only about 10 percent will die quickly and unexpectedly.[5] That suggests that 90 percent of us will require end-of-life healthcare decisions. It also means that 90 percent of us will have the time and opportunity to take control by developing a plan for the end of our life.

3. Up to 50 percent of us will require someone to make healthcare choices on our behalf at some time in our lives.

A *CNN Health* posting stated that 50 percent of patients are unable to make their own end-of-life decisions.[6] One contributing factor is that the majority of patients in Intensive Care Units are too sedated or sick to make or communicate their own wishes.[7] A study published in April 2010 by the *New England Journal of Medicine* found that approximately 30 percent of patients studied required a healthcare decision to be made on their behalf.[8]

4. The number of elderly suffering with dementia (loss of mental capability) and/or frailty is increasing.

One in eight people age sixty-five and over will be diagnosed with Alzheimer's disease. One in two—yes, 50 percent—age eighty-five and older will have Alzheimer's.[9] As the number of people living with Alzheimer's and other dementia increases, more patients will be unable to make or communicate their own treatment preferences. In fact, an estimated 40 percent of us will die after a long decline with dementia and/or frailty.[10]

5. Fewer people survive having cardiopulmonary resuscitation (C.P.R.) than you might imagine.

Robert H. Shmerling, M.D., of Beth Israel Deaconess Medical Center and associate professor at Harvard Medical School, reports that C.P.R. is effective for:[11]

- Only 2–30 percent of recipients when administered outside of the hospital,

- Only 6–15 percent of hospitalized patients,

• Fewer than 5 percent of elderly victims with multiple medical problems.

Another study demonstrated that 80 percent of cardiac arrests occur at home, and of these, 90 percent result in death. Of those who survive, over half have permanent brain damage.[12]

TV medical-related shows have led us to think people always recover. Not so. The startling reality is that very, very few people leave the hospital after receiving C.P.R. Dr. Ken Murray, Clinical Associate Professor of Family Medicine at the University of Southern California, has written that of the hundreds of people he has treated in the emergency room after getting C.P.R., only one (a healthy man with no heart trouble) walked out of the hospital. Dr. Murray says, "If a patient suffers from severe illness, old age, or a terminal disease, the odds of a good outcome from C.P.R. are infinitesimal, while the odds of suffering are overwhelming."[13]

Given these statistics, are there circumstances in which you might choose to avoid C.P.R?

6. End-of-life health care is costly for families.

Not all care is covered by Medicare or private insurance. Statistics show unexpected healthcare costs are one of the most common triggers for filing personal bankruptcy.[14] Unlike most major purchases in our lives, we have no idea what expenses we will incur for healthcare treatment, making it difficult to define any financial limits for end-of-life care.

7. End-of-life health care is costly for our country.

In a January 2010 article entitled "Choices at the End of Life," author Lisa Zamosky states: "The Centers for Medicare and Medicaid Services estimate that 5 percent of the beneficiaries who die each year take up 30 percent of the $446-billion annual Medicare budget. About 80 percent of that money is spent during the final month, on mechanical ventilators, resuscitation, and other aggressive life-sustaining care. Often, the aggressive steps taken to save someone's life are futile."[15]

8. Dying in one's home is no longer the default process.

About 80 percent of Americans die in institutions.[16] Twenty percent of deaths occur in Intensive Care Units.[17] If visiting hours are over, loved ones often die alone. In one poll, approximately 85 percent of Americans stated a desire to die at home.[18] It requires advance planning to ensure your wishes will be followed, particularly if you prefer to spend your final days and hours in your home.

9. The majority of people want to allow a more natural death.

A variety of studies indicate most Americans prefer a more natural death. Unfortunately, society has ceased to recognize dying as a natural process, treating it instead as a sickness to be overcome. Every day, thousands of dying patients across the country are transported to the emergency room in a vain attempt to cure their decline. Hospitals and physicians often assume patients want to extend their life and are, therefore, reluctant to disclose the possible negative outcomes of treatments. Doctors have difficulty acknowledging a patient is actively dying. Families make decisions without all the facts, often pursuing treatment instead of allowing a natural death to occur.

10. Most people want *some* care.

Less than 10 percent of patients refuse all care.[19] Allowing a more natural death does not mean *no* treatment. Most want *some* treatment. How "some" is defined is unique to each individual. Your definition of "some" must be clearly understood by those who could make a healthcare decision on your behalf at some point in your life.

11. Only about a third of Americans have written down their end-of-life care preferences.

A 2006 study performed by Pew Research Center for the People & the Press[20] revealed that only 29 percent of Americans have written a living will. The Hastings Center reports that number is between 15–20 percent.[21] Of those who have a written document, about one third admit they don't know where the document is located.

In Summary

Dr. Ira Byock, an expert in the field of end-of-life health care, stated on National Public Radio that an end-of-life conversation is considered by most as "always too soon, until it is too late." Let's be honest; most of us avoid this topic. But in order to move forward, we first need to recognize reality. We will all die. Remember: only 10 percent of us will die quickly and unexpectedly.[22] We all need to ask ourselves: If I'm in the remaining 90 percent, *will I be prepared and have a good death,* according to my wishes?

Take heart. Read on and use this book to help you chart a positive course. In the following chapters, you will come to understand the value of a healthcare directive. You will learn how to write a comprehensive document that ensures you receive the care you desire while supporting your loved ones as they love and support you through the dying process. Not only will you feel a tremendous sense of accomplishment and peace, you may also inspire others to follow your example.

3

Clearing Up Confusion: Why So Many Different Terms?

One of the challenges we face in discussing end-of-life issues is the interchangeable and often misunderstood terminology. All fifty states have many differences in the documents and terms that are used to reflect end-of-life preferences. Misconceptions abound. The resulting confusion has contributed to the rather low usage and poor understanding of the legal documents that have been readily available for more than forty years.

Many have asked whether healthcare reform legislation will propel us towards a national standard, thereby eliminating the variations among states. The consensus is no. Individual states will continue to own the rules that govern healthcare directives, in large part, because this is a deeply personal decision; matters of personal choice are typically governed by state law, not federal law.

The information in this chapter gives clarity to the essential words and concepts of healthcare directives, and is offered as a resource to the reader to encourage better understanding. For a comprehensive list of terms, access the glossary at the back of the book. If you are familiar with the terms, jump ahead to the next chapter.

History and Terminology

Let's get oriented with a bit of history and the myriad terms involved.

- The person writing the healthcare directive is referred to as the *principal*. For example, you are the principal for your own directive. Your mother is the principal for her own directive.

- The term *advance care planning* or **A.C.P.** has emerged in the past decade. It reflects the opportunity to proactively consider end-of-life choices in order to direct treatment in the future. Advance care planning strives to engage individuals in a process that honors one's life. Through conversation with a trained facilitator (typically arranged through the hospital or treating physician), A.C.P. helps an individual to discuss personal values, wishes, and beliefs as a framework for potential end-of-life treatment decisions. Sometimes families share in this conversation. Though not exclusively, A.C.P. is most often used with a patient who is nearing the end of life. While the result of advance care planning is most commonly a written advance healthcare directive, the clarifying conversation that can occur with loved ones can be just as valuable.

- An *advance directive* is a legal document that expresses the principal's healthcare wishes if he becomes unable to make or communicate his own decisions. Many states have adopted the term *healthcare directive* instead of advance directive. Some states use *advance healthcare directive* to capture the broadest meaning of the document. This book uses the term healthcare directive.

While a healthcare directive typically applies to end-of-life circumstances, it can also be invoked if the principal is temporarily incapacitated or unable to communicate.

A healthcare directive can include one or more of the following parts, each of which is defined in this chapter:

- Healthcare instructions (or living will)
- Durable healthcare power of attorney
- P.O.L.S.T.
- D.N.R.
- D.N.I.

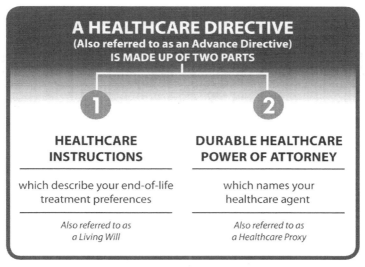

A HEALTHCARE DIRECTIVE
(Also referred to as an Advance Directive)
IS MADE UP OF TWO PARTS

1

HEALTHCARE INSTRUCTIONS

which describe your end-of-life treatment preferences

Also referred to as a Living Will

2

DURABLE HEALTHCARE POWER OF ATTORNEY

which names your healthcare agent

Also referred to as a Healthcare Proxy

Most directives include two parts

• *Healthcare instructions* broadly express the principal's preferences, including medical and non-medical wishes for end-of-life care. Instructions can include the treatments the principal wants to receive, as well as the treatments to be withheld or withdrawn in a given situation. Healthcare instructions have been adopted by many states instead of the living will.

NOTE: Though the terms living will and healthcare instructions are often used interchangeably, they are technically different document types.

- The *living will* was introduced in 1969 and was the first end-of-life document to be developed. This document reflects the principal's wishes for end-of-life medical care, usually by stating any treatment the principal wants to have withheld or withdrawn in certain circumstances. Therefore, many states have chosen to adopt healthcare instructions as part of the healthcare directive instead of a living will, because the instructions reflect a broader perspective on desired care.

- In a *durable healthcare power of attorney,* the principal appoints the person(s) who are authorized to make medical decisions on her behalf. The authority given is limited to healthcare decisions, and is used only if the principal is unable to make or communicate her own healthcare wishes.

- A *healthcare agent* is the person named by the principal in the durable healthcare power of attorney part of the health-care directive. A healthcare agent has the legal authority to make healthcare decisions for the principal when the principal lacks decision-making capacity. Of note:

  – Most often, the healthcare agent is a loved one, such as a spouse, partner, adult child, or sibling. However, in some cases, it may be a friend, attorney, pastor or colleague.

- Typically, the principal names a primary healthcare agent and one or two alternate agents. Selecting at least one alternate is highly recommended, and is suggested in most forms.

- If decisions are required on your behalf, having one agent make decisions is advisable, as opposed to requiring two agents to share this authority, and having to agree on what is best for you.

- Therefore, the term healthcare agent in the singular form is used most often in this book for the sake of simplicity when referring to the decision-maker. However, given that you should choose a primary and at least one alternate agent, all explanations and recommendations that relate to your health-care agent may actually apply to two or possibly three individuals.

- Multiple terms are used for individuals who can make medical decisions on behalf of the principal. Unfortunately, many terms, such as healthcare agent, healthcare proxy, healthcare surrogate, healthcare representative, designated patient advocate, and guardian are used interchangeably by states, in literature, and in various legal documents. See *"healthcare proxy"* in the glossary for a broader discussion of healthcare proxies and the terms noted above.

- *Decision-making capacity* (sometimes referred to as competence) is the ability to understand and make medical decisions for oneself. Typically, this means the patient must be able to understand information about the treatment decision, use the information rationally, appreciate the consequences, and communicate a decision. The process to determine a patient's level of competence usually involves evaluation by the attending doctor, and a psychiatrist or licensed psychologist. The evaluation is usually placed in the patient's medical chart.

• A *financial power of attorney* is a separate legal document that allows the principal to appoint a person who can make financial decisions and complete financial transactions on the principal's behalf. The authority given in this document is limited to financial matters only.

• A *Physician Orders for Life-Sustaining Treatment,* or *P.O.L.S.T.,* is a written physician's order for end-of-life medical treatment. The P.O.L.S.T. was developed through doctors' grassroots efforts to better address end-of-life care. Emergency personnel and nursing home staff are required to adhere to the instructions when presented with the signed document because they convey medical orders and are signed by a physician. Chapter 7 provides more detail about the P.O.L.S.T. Paradigm, and when it is appropriate to use. Because this type of document evolved through the efforts of multiple states, various titles have been adopted:

   – *M.O.L.S.T.* for Medical Orders for Life-Sustaining Treatment

   – *C.O.L.S.T.* for Clinical Orders for Life-Sustaining Treatment

   – *P.O.S.T.* for Physician Orders for Scope of Treatment

   – *M.O.S.T.* for Medical Orders for Scope of Treatment

• *Do Not Resuscitate,* or *D.N.R.,* is a written doctor's order that indicates the patient does not want to be resuscitated if his heart stops beating or he stops breathing. D.N.R. means the medical team should not attempt cardiopulmonary resuscitation (C.P.R.), intubation (ventilation), internal or external stimulation of the heart, or administer medications to stimulate the heart. The term D.N.A.R. is preferred by many where the "A" indicates "attempt." **Do Not Attempt Resuscitation** more accurately indicates that C.P.R. and other medical procedures are performed to *attempt* to resuscitate the patient and may or may not succeed. Chapter 7 provides more detail about the D.N.R. order.

- **Do Not Intubate,** or **D.N.I.,** is a written doctor's order that indicates the patient does not want to receive intubation if he stops breathing. This means the patient does not want to have a tube inserted through his airway and attached to a ventilator that mechanically breathes for him. Chapter 7 provides more detail about the D.N.I. order.

- **Cardiopulmonary resuscitation,** or **C.P.R.,** involves procedures and medications to restart and stabilize a person's heart and breathing. C.P.R. can include chest compressions, electrical stimulation to the heart, and other procedures or medication to restart the heart or maintain its rhythm. It may also include rescue or artificial breathing using intubation (ventilation) to reduce the risk of brain injury due to lack of oxygen.

- In 1990, Congress passed the **Patient Self-Determination Act.** This federal law requires healthcare facilities to elicit and honor a patient's healthcare directive to the extent required by state law. Whether patients have the right to accept or refuse medical treatment of any kind is determined by state law.

In Summary

The myriad terms noted above contribute to a veil of confusion for many individuals. Simply stated, a healthcare directive can include end-of-life healthcare instructions, and/or name a healthcare agent. Doctor's orders, such as a P.O.L.S.T, D.N.R. or D.N.I. can also be considered important elements of a thorough healthcare directive, particularly for those who may be very near to the end of life.

4

Ten Reasons to Write
a Thorough Healthcare Directive

Are you a planner? The idea of writing down your end-of-life wishes might make total sense to you. Perhaps you are familiar with end-of-life issues, or have been touched by the bad death of a loved one or friend, and therefore you recognize the value of expressing your preferences. You believe writing a healthcare directive is **something you need to do for yourself.**

But what if planning is not your cup of tea? It may help to frame end-of-life preparation differently. Consider a healthcare directive as a loving gift to your family and friends. Recognize that your courage and your willingness to address your mortality will undoubtedly **ease the sadness and the difficult decisions your loved ones will face** at the end of your life.

Top Ten Reasons

Ten reasons should compel each of us to write a directive.

Do it for you.

Approach the end of life with greater control and less fear.

1. Receive all the care—and only the care—you desire.

2. Make decisions while you are able.

3. Live your life—prepared.

Do it for those you love, and who love you.

Give them peace of mind.

  4. Be proactive if you don't want to be a burden.

  5. Confront the myth that they will know what to do.

  6. Protect and maintain family harmony.

  7. Preserve family assets.

  8. Help your loved ones let go.

  9. Keep decisions within your private circle of loved ones.

  10. Legally empower your chosen healthcare agent.

Reason 1: Receive all the care—and only the care—you desire.

To ensure your treatment preferences are followed:

- Communicate in writing what treatments you *do* and *do not* want to receive.

- Manage the healthcare system; take charge.

- Prepare your healthcare agent and loved ones to honor your wishes.

Communicate in writing what treatments you do and do not want to receive.

In order to communicate your treatment preferences, you must first wrestle with your own thoughts and feelings to determine what end-of-life health care makes sense to you. Many individuals offer vague generalities either verbally or even in writing, such as:

- "I don't want to receive extraordinary or heroic measures."

- "I don't want any invasive treatments."

- "I don't want to be hooked up to machines."

- "When the time has come, just let me go."

Such statements are woefully inadequate, and really challenge those making decisions for you to try to determine what you mean. What you deem extraordinary or invasive might be considered standard treatment to someone else. Asking someone to determine "when the time has come" to let you go is a tremendous responsibility, if not a burden. Your specific instructions are needed.

Heroic or extraordinary measures can include cardiopulmonary resuscitation (C.P.R.), trauma surgery (outside of an operating room), dialysis, and high doses of antibiotics or chemotherapy. It can also include any other medication or procedure that could have a high risk of causing damage to the patient, yet without which death is certain.

Your intention could be to receive all possible care, even knowing the risks. Or you could prefer to allow nature to take its course. Most individuals take the middle road and choose limited care. That requires an individual definition for limited. Limited could include or exclude any number of treatments or procedures, such as antibiotics, dialysis, blood transfusion, implants (pacemaker), surgery, psychotropic drugs, or other medications. Be more specific in describing your wishes. For example, if you don't want to be on a ventilator, is it because of the loss of mobility or independence? Do you fear an inability to communicate? Would a ventilator be okay for a few days, but not for numerous months? Write a specific statement, e.g., "I do not wish to be on a ventilator because . . ."

Phrases like "no heroic measures" or "limited care" do not directly define your wishes. Clearly articulating in writing the level of medical intervention you desire is your right, opportunity, and responsibility.

Manage the healthcare system; take charge.

Recognize that you or your healthcare agent may meet resistance from your medical team if you choose to limit your care or allow a natural death. You or your agent could be pushed to pursue undesired treatments. Be prepared to push back and take charge.

Our healthcare system is built on the principle of keeping patients alive. Doctors are trained and, by nature of their profession, desire to save you. Our cultural propensity for lawsuits has backed our healthcare providers into a corner; they'd better do everything possible to save you, or they might be sued for malpractice, particularly when family members disagree about a loved one's care. Some doctors have a "savior complex," believing one more treatment or one more procedure might be the cure. Moreover, they do not want a patient to die on their watch. They hold out hope for you and your family even if the odds are tiny. And, of course, miracles do happen.

Acknowledging death is a difficult conversation for anyone, including doctors. Few physicians have been trained how to openly concede a patient is dying. Amazingly, some are unfamiliar with the signs of the dying process, instead perceiving these signs as symptoms that require treatment. Patients and loved ones could be left wondering what is really happening. Often, patients ask the nurse, "Am I dying?" after the doctor has made a quick exit.

C.P.R.

Many people consider C.P.R. and ventilation invasive, particularly for patients who are frail. C.P.R. compressions can cause bruising or fracture of the ribs or sternum. Broken ribs can puncture a lung, liver and/or the spleen. If C.P.R. is not correctly administered, or is started too late, brain damage can result.

C.P.R. was originally conceived by a pediatrician who was striving to restart the heart of an otherwise healthy child. Over time, C.P.R. has become a standard of care in most situations, even with terminally ill patients or the very elderly. It can be traumatic for the patient and for loved ones standing by. Quite recently, some hospitals have begun to evaluate their approach to C.P.R., choosing to be less aggressive in administering invasive treatments for patients who are actively dying and have very little chance of surviving the procedure.

While survival rates are low (listed in chapter 2), C.P.R. can sometimes successfully restart the patient's heart rhythm and breathing. Survivors are understandably grateful for bystanders or physicians who work to restart their heart.

> Without knowing that their loved one is actively dying, families often pursue treatment that is not wanted or even needed.

Unwanted and unnecessary care has a cost. The financial component is real. Like it or not, and this can sound crass, our healthcare system is built on a fee-for-service model. The more services rendered, the more fees received. Doctors and hospitals have a financial incentive to give us *more* care, even when such care has little to no chance of prolonging a meaningful life. Hospitals are a supply-side business. They need to fill their beds in order to make payroll. Additionally, practicing defensive medicine to avoid litigation adds to the cost of end-of-life care.

In fairness, the healthcare delivery industry is striving to implement financial reform. Healthcare economics is a complex issue. In response to the particularly high cost of end-of-life health care, many proactive hospitals have trained physicians to more actively engage the healthcare agent and loved ones in discussing medically appropriate treatment for a dying patient. Some hospitals offer palliative care specialists who are physicians trained to address patients' symptoms and pain to prevent needless suffering and unnecessary treatment. Palliative care specialists are particularly adept at facilitating conversation with patients and loved ones as they cope with the reality of the end of life.

Equally real is the insurance industry's role in containing costs. Your healthcare agent and whomever you empower to manage your financial matters may be required to take on your insurance company to secure coverage for expensive treatments. If treatment costs were not covered, would that change your wishes? That's a question you will want to consider when creating your healthcare directive.

Add to this, advances in technology. Did you know it is now possible to replicate nearly every major bodily function? Your heart, lungs, kidneys, and even your liver can be managed with machines outside of your body. Nutrition and hydration can be artificially administered through tubes. In certain cases, a patient can be kept alive for months or even years. Sadly, many patients receive undesired heroic measures, leading to long stays in Intensive Care, hooked up to machines.

While it may be possible to extend life, the profoundly individual question remains: Where is the line between extending life and prolonging the dying process for you?

> Entrust end-of-life decisions to a healthcare agent who will advocate for your stated wishes, even if facing opposition to a physician's recommendation.

Prepare your healthcare agent and loved ones to honor your wishes.

Anticipate the difficulty a healthcare agent will face if required to make life-or-death decisions on your behalf. You want every assurance that your agent will not revoke your decisions under duress. Your healthcare agent could have to withhold or withdraw treatment according to your wishes, in spite of the objections of well-meaning loved ones or healthcare providers. Alternatively, your agent may need to advocate for additional treatment, even if others perceive the treatment as futile. Your best defense is a good offense. Communicate your end-of-life healthcare wishes through a written healthcare directive. Then, conduct a family meeting to explain your decisions. Pointedly ask that your wishes be honored. You could even have loved ones sign your directive to indicate their commitment to abide by your preferences.

> Anticipate resistance from loved ones.
> The best defense is a good offense.
> Use your voice before you lose your choice.

Reason 2: Make decisions while you are able.

As more people live into their eighties and nineties, more individuals live with dementia, defined as the loss of mental or cognitive capability due to changes in brain function. Dementia is marked by significant memory loss and often a change in personality. It can be caused by brain disease or injury. Alzheimer's, Parkinson's, strokes, and traumatic brain injury are commonly recognized causes of dementia. Projections show 40 percent of us will die after a long, slow journey through dementia and/or frailty.[23]

The ethical challenge lies in discerning a person's cognitive ability to make his own decisions.

- How can you ethically discuss end-of-life decisions with a loved one with dementia?

- How can you be at peace, wondering if the words they speak are really their heartfelt wishes, or perhaps confused or influenced by a well-intended loved one or medical professional?

As our family experienced with Mom, dementia is insidious. Good days are followed by bad days. We could have had a seemingly normal conversation about Mom's end-of-life wishes on a good day. But within a few days, Mom's behavior would manifest the reality of her dementia. When is it too late for a person with dementia to voice end-of-life preferences?

The backlash from the "death-panel" phrase bantered about by the 2008 political pundits rightfully raised awareness of the ethical hazards for end-of-life treatment. Pro-life advocates appropriately voiced concern that elderly, vulnerable adults with disabilities, and those with dementia, can be pressured into signing a D.N.R. order or a healthcare directive that fore-goes treatment. Recording end-of-life wishes while you are mentally and physically able is imperative. If you should ever be unable to understand your options, make informed choices, or communicate your wishes, your written healthcare directive will protect you.

Plan for healthcare decisions while you are mentally capable.

Reason 3: Live your life—prepared.

One of the first things I learned about my husband when we started dating was his childhood history as a Boy Scout. "Be prepared" is one of the Boy Scouts' mottos. When we feel prepared in life—whether for something enjoyable or for a challenge—we approach it with greater confidence.

The emergency room is not conducive to clear thinking. Panic and emotion overtake logic. When pressed for urgent decisions, families typically adopt the default approach of requesting all possible care without anticipating the conse-quences of this choice.

Though we cannot control all the circumstances at the end of life, a plan helps us anticipate the possibilities and pre-determine our response. A plan gives us cause to pause, and creates a sense of control. Reflecting in advance makes choices less emotionally charged during a crisis. Anxiety and fear are subdued by a thoughtful plan. Heightened emotions can be more effectively managed when decisions about end-of-life care have been reached calmly.

> Be prepared with a written plan for your healthcare choices. Defining your preferences in advance reduces anxiety and fear in a crisis.

Reason 4: Be proactive if you don't want to be a burden.

Perhaps the most frequently uttered phrase by aging adults is the statement: "I don't want to be a burden." We loathe the prospect of burdening our loved ones with our care. In spite of our best efforts, we will likely need care from, and have to rely on, our loved ones.

Make your expectations clear. This works in both directions. By that, I mean you might wish to be cared for by loved ones, or, you could prefer the safety and social interaction of assisted living if you are unable to live independently and remain in your home.

Perhaps you expect to be cared for indefinitely by loved ones, knowing that you would do the same for them. By having a conversation now about your expectations, your family can consider how personal care could be delivered in your home or theirs. Funds could be set aside to address physical changes to the home's environment, such as adding handrails to a shower or accommodating a wheelchair. Possibly through such conversations, you will discover concerns that could be discussed now, and in doing so, reduce the stress loved ones might experience in the future. If feasible, funds might also be set aside to supplement the income of those caring for you. Families often experience significant financial strain if they need to step away from their employment in order to serve as a caregiver, so it is better if the financial considerations are addressed early.

Alternatively, it is possible your fierce independence and pride makes the prospect of being cared for by loved ones unthinkable. Maybe you have a strong sense of boundaries, or perhaps you do not wish to experience any sense of indebtedness. You might actually prefer the care received through a quality nursing home or long-term care facility. For you, this is the most dignified option, giving you the strongest sense of control.

Or perhaps, you are deeply concerned about the physical, financial, emotional, and spiritual toll your loved ones would experience as caregivers. Maybe your concern for their needs takes precedence in your decision; your wish to preserve their quality of life is most important to you. Communicate your preference to receive care at a safe, clean, well-run assisted-living facility. Remove any future guilt your loved ones might feel by choosing to relocate you if you are no longer able to care for yourself at home. In fact, you might develop a plan to proactively

> What if I should follow in my mother's footsteps, and develop Alzheimer's disease? I have asked my husband to move me to a safe, caring, and comfortable facility after no more than a year of care in our home. That is my personal view of not being a burden.

seek some level of assistance in the future, rather than waiting for a crisis to force a sudden change in living arrangements.

> None of us knows what circumstances are likely to befall us. We don't want to be a burden, yet more than likely we will need assistance in our elder years. Talking about your expectations now is an act of love. So, too, is financial preparation.

Reason 5: Confront the myth that they will know what to do.

Even if your spouse or adult child knows you well, imagine the emotional stress they might experience if a doctor asked them to quickly make a life-or-death decision regarding your healthcare treatment. Young couples rarely speak about end-of-life decisions, assuming the topic can wait. A tragic accident occurs, and a twenty-something husband is confronted with an impossible decision with no idea what his pregnant wife would want. If you are older, perhaps you've talked about end-of-life treatment. But what if that conversation occurred a dozen years ago? Or what if, during the incredibly painful moment of trying to reach a decision, your loved one wonders if you might feel differently due to recent circumstances in your life? For most human beings, intense emotional stress makes it nearly impossible to think clearly or to remember a distant conversation. Finally, if you've never had the conversation, recognize that your loved one could project personal wishes for care into the situation. This is a natural and common tendency for us all.

Some interesting research reveals that a high level of deep depression frequently occurs with those who had to make a life-and-death decision for a loved one when the patient's wishes were not certain. Post-traumatic stress disorder (P.T.S.D.) can even result. Imagine the anguish of second-guessing the decision in addition to the natural pain of grieving for the loss of a loved one.

Remove this ambiguity not only by having the conversation about end-of-life choices, but also by recording your wishes in writing. Continue the conversation throughout your life. Review your directive every couple of years; refresh your decisions, and update your document as necessary to ensure it accurately reflects your wishes. Have a conversation with loved ones any time you update your wishes in your directive.

Never assume your loved ones will know your preferences. The intense emotional stress of a crisis makes it nearly impossible to think clearly or to remember past conversations about the end of life. Put your choices in writing.

Reason 6: Protect and maintain family harmony.

Family members frequently disagree on the appropriate treatment for a loved one. Some members might believe their loved one will be saved through aggressive treatment. Others recoil at the thought of invasive treatment for a frail loved one, feeling the time has come to let go and allow a more peaceful passing. Without your clear instructions, your loved ones could face tremendous turmoil, even leading to permanently damaged family relationships. In more extreme cases, lawsuits can ensue. What a painful legacy to leave—family members estranged when they need each other most to cope with grieving your loss. Instead, leave a legacy of family unity.

Imagine the magnified intensity of such conflict in blended families. For example, what if the adult children disagree with the stepmother regarding the care for their father? Given the prevalence of blended families in our society, the potential for such conflict is enormous. If you are part of a blended family, your loved ones can be particularly susceptible to the hazards of end-of-life conflict, especially when **your own firm voice** isn't being clearly heard through a written healthcare directive. Be courageous—have the conversation now. Make sure all parties understand your selection for a healthcare agent. In some circumstances, it might be wise to appoint both the spouse from a current marriage, with one or more of the adult children from an earlier marriage. In that case, be certain to give final decision-making authority to one person. If adult children will not be involved in the decision-making, let them know now, and explain why. Don't make your current spouse have to defend her or his healthcare decisions on your behalf to adult children from a former marriage.

> Promote family harmony and unity, particularly during a time of stress and grief. Clearly explain your end-of-life healthcare choices to avoid the possibility of conflict between loved ones who may disagree about your treatment.

Reason 7: Preserve family assets.

Health care is costly. While private insurance or Medicare covers many costs, most patients face out-of-pocket costs for their co-pay, or for services and supplies that are not covered. A recent TV commercial shows a husband packing a final box, then walking away from a beautiful home. In the next scene, he is unpacking boxes in a tiny apartment. In the closing scene, he walks into a nursing home to visit his wife. It is a poignant depiction of what happens to many families when finances are drained through costly end-of-life care.

Unanticipated healthcare expenses are a leading cause of bankruptcy. One study found that 40 percent of families became impoverished due to the financial cost of providing care for a terminally ill loved one.[24] A study conducted by the Health Care Financing Administration (renamed the Centers for Medicare & Medicaid Services), recorded that one-third of terminally ill patients with insurance used up most, or all, of their savings to cover uninsured medical expenses.[25]

In a story presented by CBS's *60 Minutes,* originally aired in 2009, research indicated that Medicare paid $50 billion in 2008 for doctor and hospital bills during the final two months of patients' lives, 20–30 percent of which had no meaningful impact on the patient's health. In the segment, Dr. Ira Byock, Director of Palliative Care at the Dartmouth-Hitchcock Medical Center, noted that it costs up to $10,000 per day to maintain a patient in the Intensive Care Unit (I.C.U.). "This is the way so many Americans die. Something like 18 to 20 percent of Americans spend their last days in an I.C.U.," Dr. Byock told *60 Minutes* reporter Steve Kroft. "And, you know, it's extremely expensive. It's uncomfortable. Many times they have to be sedated so that they don't reflexively pull out a tube, or sometimes their hands are restrained. This is not the way most people would want to spend their last days of life. And yet this has become almost the medical last rites for people as they die."

Many families invest thousands of dollars to protect their family's financial assets through an estate plan and will. However, rarely do we consider how our end-of-life healthcare choices could financially affect those we love most. Families might suffer enormous financial loss, even bankruptcy, due to end-of-life health care—care that your loved one, in fact, might not even want.

This delicate subject of financial limits for end-of-life treatment is deeply personal. Nonetheless, I raise the question. Would you choose to set any financial boundaries for the care you receive?

> End-of-life health care is costly, and not all expenses are covered by insurance. Consider the financial implications for your loved ones when deciding on your end-of-life choices.

Reason 8: Help your loved ones let go.

Often, the dying process is prolonged because loved ones are unable to let go. Prior to the intense emotions of a crisis, convey your personal feelings about extending life versus prolonging death. The line between those two is very gray and deeply personal.

Practical questions to consider include:

- Is it important to you that you be kept alive until your family members have all gathered?

- Is it important to them, for their sense of closure, to be physically present even if that requires keeping you alive for a period of time?

- What would be an acceptable period of time to wait—a couple of days, a week?

- Just how far should treatment go to keep you alive until family can gather?

While technology affords 24/7 connection through electronic communication, we live in a far less relational world. We ache for closeness. Many families are distant and fractured. Often a dying patient is kept alive so others can come to the bedside to make peace.

Rather than wait until a crisis, consider how you might reach out now to strengthen and mend family relationships. Find joy in living with deeper relationships in the present.

Additionally, the dying process has become unfamiliar and unrecognized to many of us. Your loved ones may need to be reminded to look for, recognize, and honor the signs of the dying process. Ask your physician to coach them. In *OK to Die*,[26] authors Kristian Murphy and E.R. physician Dr. Monica Williams-Murphy write:

Unless one dies suddenly, there is usually a slow, step-by-step progression downward in energy, vitality, appetite, wits, mentality, and wakefulness. The tempo of this step-by-step progression can also vary, occurring over years, months, or sometimes, just days. Many family members really expect that an eighty-nine-year-old person who is taking these downward steps can be rehabilitated, or given medications, which will enable that loved one to start taking steps back upward toward becoming their previous selves. They often expect them to become more energetic, more awake, more interactive, and so forth. Occasionally, this does happen, but it is the rare occasion, it is only a short reprieve from the inevitable.

Proactively address the emotions of loved ones through clear instructions in your healthcare directive. They may need your help to let you go.

Reason 9: Keep decisions within your private circle of loved ones.

Years ago, the media covered the Terri Schiavo case. It made the headlines because it demonstrated an extreme. Terri's husband and parents battled over her care after she entered into a vegetative state in 1990 at the age of twenty-six. Terri's husband believed she would not want to continue receiving artificially administered food and fluids in her persistent vegetative state. Her parents vehemently disagreed, arguing for all possible care to be administered indefinitely. Years of court battles ensued. While it's uncommon to reach that height of national visibility, too often circumstances occur that find family members facing off legally. Besides the legal issues and cost, medical decisions for your care can be left to hospital administrators, a judge, or a court-appointed guardian when a healthcare agent has not been properly appointed and legally recorded in writing.

Keep the decision-making private. Avoid legal battles. Write your healthcare directive to expressly define your preferences and choice of agent.

Reason 10: Legally empower your chosen healthcare agent.

What if the person you would appoint as your healthcare agent is not a relative? In that case, if you have not made that appointment *legally binding* through a durable healthcare power of attorney, your preferred decision-maker will not be legally empowered to act on your behalf as your healthcare agent.

- Assuring your choice for healthcare agent is legally binding is particularly relevant for those in a long-term relationship, but not legally married. In many cases, estranged parents or siblings have greater legal authority to make healthcare decisions on your behalf than your lifelong partner.

- Some individuals choose to appoint a close friend, attorney, or other non-relative to the role of healthcare agent.

  – For example, a spouse may not have the emotional capacity to make difficult end-of-life decisions. It could be most loving to ask a more objective, yet trusted person to shoulder this burden.

  – For any number of reasons, parents might wish to avoid choosing any one child as a healthcare agent, preferring instead to engage a close friend.

  – Consider choosing a friend or sibling as a first alternate healthcare agent, in case both you and your spouse are involved in an accident at the same time.

- Through your healthcare directive, you can also declare who should *not* participate in your healthcare decisions. This can be particularly useful in some situations, and several examples are provided in chapter 8.

> Next-of-kin relatives are the default surrogate if a healthcare agent is not legally specified. Legally empower the person **you** choose to serve as your healthcare agent by writing your healthcare directive.

In Summary

The ten reasons for writing your healthcare directive demonstrate the multi-dimensional nature of preparing for the end of life. The **medical** dimension is central to the decisions you will make as you express your preference for the level of intervention and care you wish to receive. By nature, a healthcare directive is a **legal** instrument, incorporating legal power to act on your behalf through your appointment of a healthcare agent. Grappling with end of life touches our **emotional** core, requiring decisions to be made from the heart. Moreover, the **social** dimension—how our decisions will impact those we love—calls us to stretch our thinking beyond our own needs. **Financial** considerations may influence decisions. And for many, the **spiritual** dimension is the most important. Preparing for the end of life calls forth personal, sacred reflection.

This chapter is written to convince you of the merits of writing and communicating your healthcare directive. I trust you're inspired and now you can inspire loved ones and friends to do the same. By writing and communicating our healthcare directives, we can mitigate and even eliminate future suffering by ensuring comfort care is advocated according to our wishes. We can protect our loved ones from the stress and anguish of making decisions without our instructions. Finally, we can limit the spending of healthcare dollars to only **desired** end-of-life treatment.

Now that you understand why you need to express your end-of-life healthcare preferences in writing, it's time to move on and learn what should be included to create a meaningful healthcare directive.

WHAT

What should I include in my healthcare directive?

Define what "quality of life" means to you.

Guide treatment decisions by sharing your values and beliefs. Describe what makes life meaningful for you.

Write clear healthcare instructions.

Communicate your treatment preferences to ensure you receive all the care—and only the care—you desire.

Choose your healthcare agents.

Name the people who should make decisions on your behalf if you are unable to do so.

Support your loved ones.

Share messages with loved ones that communicate your personal needs for support and remembrance.

5

What Documents Do You Need?

Every adult should write a healthcare directive. By now you are hopefully convinced, even encouraged, to document your end-of-life preferences. Optimally, you are willing to describe your healthcare decisions in writing to be certain your wishes are clear, and you have at least one person you can trust to serve as your healthcare agent.

However, not everyone has the optimal situation. For some, there really is no one trustworthy enough to serve as a healthcare agent. Others may be physically, mentally, or emotionally unwilling or unable to write down their preferences.

Recall from chapter 3 that a healthcare directive typically has two parts: healthcare instructions and a healthcare power of attorney. The three scenarios that are presented in this chapter demonstrate that in some cases, only one of the two parts is completed. Assess your situation to determine which parts should comprise your healthcare directive. If you are uncertain how to proceed, consult with an attorney.

Scenario #1: You are willing and able to write down your preferences, and you have at least one person you can trust as your agent.

Write a complete healthcare directive.
This is the most comprehensive approach, and is highly recommended. It offers the greatest likelihood that your wishes will be honored. This approach includes both your healthcare instructions and the durable healthcare power of attorney that names your healthcare agent and alternate(s).

Scenario #2: You are unable or unwilling to write down your preferences, but you have at least one person you can trust as your agent.

Write only a durable healthcare power of attorney to express your selection of a healthcare agent. This is appropriate if you are unwilling or unable to write down your instructions. You may prefer to verbally express your preferences, or you may simply trust that your selected agent will make decisions in your best interest.

Recognize that this approach can add tremendous stress for your healthcare agent. Consider taking the time to write down your instructions and complete an entire healthcare directive (approach for scenario #1). If you are unable to write or type your wishes, consider using a tape recorder and having your recording transcribed into your healthcare directive. Numerous transcription services are available via the Internet.

Scenario #3: You are willing and able to write down your preferences, but you have no one you can trust as your agent.

Write only your healthcare instructions.

Your instructions state what kinds of treatments you want to receive and treatments you want to refuse in various circumstances. If you do not have a person you fully trust to name as your agent, you should carefully write down your instructions so the medical professionals treating you will know your preferences. In this case, it is imperative that your physician receives a copy of your directive so that your treatment preferences can be honored by your medical team at the end of life.

It is best to have a healthcare agent who can advocate on your behalf. Consider an attorney, clergy person, respected friend, neighbor, or business colleague. However, *if you do not have a trusted advocate, do not name anyone as your agent.*

Recognize that a decision-maker can be named to fill this vacuum. The attending physician could be approached by a loved one who qualifies as next-of-kin, asking to serve as your surrogate. The physician could appoint a family member to make the decisions. A court can name a guardian or conservator. If this is your circumstance, make your instructions known to your physician.

If the End Is Near

If you are facing the possibility of your passing within the next twelve months, speak with your physician about also writing doctor's orders, which may include a P.O.L.S.T. and/or a D.N.R. This is an important document that strengthens your end-of-life wishes in the form of a medical order. A referral to hospice for information should also be requested. Chapter 7 discusses these options in greater detail.

What If I Do Not Write a Healthcare Directive?

If you should be unable to make or communicate your own healthcare decisions and have not written a healthcare directive:

All life-sustaining treatment will be delivered. Without consent to do otherwise, hospitals will pursue all possible care in order to attempt to stabilize and restore you, the patient, and candidly, to avoid a lawsuit.

Someone will make the decisions. The possibilities include next-of-kin, the attending physician, hospital administrators, or a court-ordered guardian. Chapter 8 provides detailed information about these possibilities.

What If I Change My Mind?

At any time, you can change your mind by revoking your healthcare directive. I will say that again. *At any time, you can change your mind, as long as you still have the mental capacity to do so.* More than likely, your opinions about end-of-life care will change over time. What could seem unacceptable at age thirty could be quite acceptable at age eighty.

To revoke your healthcare directive, you must do one of the following:

• Destroy the document by tearing it up or shredding it.

• Direct another person to destroy it in your presence.

- Sign a written and dated statement that you want it revoked.

- State in front of two witnesses that it is revoked. This would typically occur when you are hospitalized, and you communicate your revocation to your doctor(s) and/or nurse(s).

- Execute a new healthcare directive.

Revoking your directive in writing, and then destroying any copies, provides the best protection. It is crucial that you notify your healthcare agents, your healthcare providers and anyone to whom you have given access to this document about the revocation. If you have executed a new healthcare directive, give each one a new document.

Make Your Documents Legal

Your documents must be executed to be made legal. Laws differ by state regarding what is required to execute a healthcare directive. Chapter 10 covers this step of the process in detail.

What If I Have a Home in More Than One State?

Some states, but not all, extend reciprocity to other states for healthcare directives. There's a catch. Here is an example of a hospital policy statement:

"A living will or other type of advance directive from another state, even though it does not meet the requirements of [HOME STATE], is legally valid and enforceable in [HOME STATE] if it satisfies the legal requirements of the state in which it was executed."[27]

The question then becomes: How is a physician in an emergency room supposed to evaluate whether the patient's healthcare directive document satisfies the legal requirements of the state in which it was executed? Because physicians cannot be expected to assess the legal validity of a document, some hospitals have adopted a risk-management strategy that allows only advance directives from their home state to be honored. Therefore, if you have residences in multiple states, your best protection is to have a healthcare directive for each state. They should be consistent and executed at the same time. If that's too much trouble, you can add a statement such as, "This healthcare directive is intended to be valid in any jurisdiction in which it is presented." It might help, but it is not a guarantee.

In Summary

Communicating your preferences and your choice of healthcare agent affords the best assurance that your wishes will be followed at the end of life. However, if circumstances do not allow you to complete both the healthcare instructions and the healthcare power of attorney, having at least your wishes, or your selected agent, recorded is a positive step to prepare for your final days. Finally, if you are nearing the end, having doctor's orders in the form of a P.O.L.S.T. or a D.N.R. is wise.

6

How Do *You* Define
a Meaningful Quality of Life?

Quality of life—"the degree to which a person enjoys the important possibilities of his or her life."[28] That's how the researchers at the University of Toronto's Quality of Life Research Unit define quality of life.

- What are the important possibilities of your life?

- How would you describe a marvelous day or weekend?

- When you reminisce, what memories conjure a sense of well-being, of happiness, of enjoying life?

- What gives you the greatest sense of joy and purpose?

As you consider end-of-life treatment preferences, it is helpful to describe the circumstances that, even if they mean a more modest life, would still make living well possible. As we age, most of us will experience some amount of physical, emotional, or mental decline. We will have aches and pains, possibly experience reduced memory, and we will slow down. A loss of some of our capability is a natural part of life. Nonetheless, we can adjust. We can redefine our approach to daily living. We can still pursue the important possibilities of life and live well as we adapt to physical, emotional or mental changes. The human capacity to adapt is truly remarkable.

The pressing question is whether we can articulate a point

that, when it is reached, we would welcome death. Are there circumstances in which living would no longer be tolerable? When you genuinely believe you would be unable or unwilling to adapt? Based upon my experience as the daughter of someone who lived with Alzheimer's for twenty years, I have strong opinions for my own life regarding when I would choose to cease medical care.

In order to make healthcare decisions on your behalf, your healthcare agent and your medical team need to understand what makes you tick—what makes life meaningful for you. The best-made decisions will address you as a whole person rather than make decisions that are directed merely at managing a disease or symptoms.

Quality of Life Requires Definition

Many of the living wills written in the '80s and '90s included broad and vague statements. One particularly recorded phrase then, and even now, is, "I don't want any care that will compromise the quality of my life." My father has uttered that exact phrase.

What does that mean? If faced with life-altering treatment choices for my father, how could I discern what would be acceptable to him? How would I know to decline a treatment that would render his quality of life unacceptable to him?

So, when I asked Dad what he meant, he replied, "I don't want any care that will incapacitate me." This answer was not much clearer. I kept pressing.

"What if you had all of your mental capability, but were physically limited to being in bed? What if you could no longer speak but could write your thoughts or respond by blinking or squeezing? What if you could no longer _____?"

I gave my father many "what ifs," and he patiently replied. With each reply, his definition of quality of life solidified.

For some, this train of thought may be moot. If you value life above all, even in the direst of circumstances, your healthcare directive can reflect that **any** quality of life is acceptable. You can instruct your healthcare agent and medical team to pursue **all** appropriate treatment.

How to Define Quality of Life

Defining a meaningful quality of life can seem daunting. Breaking it down into various dimensions or attributes makes it less overwhelming. For example, you could reflect on your views about the importance of your mobility for your quality of life. What if you:

- Required a wheelchair or walker to move about?
- Became homebound due to the difficulty of moving from place to place?
- Were bedridden?
- Required assistance for basic personal care and grooming due to your lack of mobility?

Other dimensions worth considering as you describe a meaningful quality of life include:

- Communication,
- Emotional and social interaction,
- Recognition of loved ones,
- Completion of daily activities, such as eating, dressing, using the toilet, and showering,
- Retention of your sense of privacy.

> Consider answering this question for the various areas that define your quality of life: "I believe I can live well, and still have an acceptable quality of life if . . ."

Here are a couple of examples from my own healthcare directive. My definition of quality of life includes the following statements, among others:

"I believe I can live well and still have an acceptable quality of life if I am able to recognize my loved ones about half of the time, if I know their names, know how we are connected, and can have pleasant conversation."

"I believe I can live well, and still have an acceptable quality of life, even if I need assistance in all my daily living needs. I accept that I could require round-the-clock care and assistance in order to eat, dress, bathe, use the toilet, and manage grooming and personal hygiene."

As you can see, I'm fine with physical limitations, but I am less accepting of memory limitations. If I become unable to recognize my loved ones, I'm ready to let nature take its course if I should have an infection or heart attack. That is my choice. What are your wishes?

Values and Beliefs

Many people find it both helpful and enriching to spend time answering broad questions that reflect their personal values and beliefs. In the same way that families pass on their financial assets through a traditional will, many choose to pass on their values through an "ethical will" and/or by including value statements in the healthcare directive. Family physician Dr. Barry Baines is Associate Medical Director for Hospice of the

Twin Cities, and also Vice President, Celebrations of Life. He writes in his book *Ethical Wills:*

> Both personally and professionally, I have become a strong proponent of the ethical will as a vehicle for clarifying and communicating the meaning in our lives to our families and communities. I strongly believe that those who wish to reflect on and share life's experience will find an ethical will a useful tool. Those who wish to examine their moral underpinnings discover it to be an excellent forum for contemplation. Those who want to be remembered authentically and for their gifts of heart, mind, and spirit take satisfaction in knowing what they hold most valued is "on the record," not to be lost or forgotten.[29]

Consider incorporating statements about your values and beliefs into your healthcare directive. Embrace the opportunity to reflect important thoughts that you hope loved ones will read, in the present (when your directive is complete and you share it), and in the future (should the need arise to make a decision on your behalf). As with the definition of a meaningful quality of life, these statements can inform and support your decision-makers during the stress of making decisions on your behalf, if such a time occurs.

For example, your healthcare directive could include reflections for any or all of the following:

- What has given you the greatest sense of purpose in your life?

- What spiritual beliefs, if any, sustain you during difficult times?

- What comfort, if any, would sharing your beliefs provide to your loved ones?

- What moral or spiritual lessons, or life wisdom, if any, do you want to pass along?

- What instructions or advice about specific life events do you want to impart to prepare your children for the future?

- What legacy do you hope to leave?

Taking the time to reflect upon and respond to these big life questions can create a marvelous opening for family dialogue. What a gift you can offer by incorporating these value statements into your healthcare directive.

In Summary

How you define living well is integral to making healthcare treatment decisions at the end of your life. Wise decisions about your care address who you are, and how you want to live. To that end, a well-written healthcare directive that incorporates how you define a meaningful quality of life offers important guidance to your decision-makers. Including your beliefs, wishes, and values will remind your medical team that you are a person with a spirit, not merely a body that is failing. Reflecting *who you are,* as part of your directive, supports *your choices* that are expressed in *your voice*.

7

Medical Decisions Are the Core of Your Healthcare Directive

It is difficult, and even frightening, to imagine ourselves in the circumstances where any end-of-life decisions would be required. Writing a healthcare directive will push you to consider and make core medical choices. I recommend reading this chapter twice.

The majority of patients that reach the emergency room with a life-threatening illness or injury have never contemplated their healthcare preferences. A crisis is certainly not the opportune moment to face these decisions for the first time. An emergency room physician must rapidly determine whether a patient's life is threatened due to a treatable, or an irreversible, condition and to administer the appropriate treatment. Urgency demands quick and decisive action.

- How would your loved ones respond under the high stress and shock of that situation?

- Could they honor your wishes? Or, more likely, would they authorize all possible treatments now, and consider the consequences later?

- Conversely, would your loved ones direct the physician to only address your symptoms and pain when you, in fact, would want to receive all possible treatments to extend your life?

- How will your loved ones or medical team know your wishes?

Remember that you may change your healthcare directive at any time. If you are able to speak for yourself, you may change your mind and communicate different choices in the midst of the health challenge.

Core Decisions

Stages of Planning

In broad brushstrokes, decisions for the end of life can occur in one of three stages of planning:

Stage One: You are healthy. You are planning proactively. Decisions are in a more abstract and hypothetical mindset.

Stage Two: You are wrestling with a serious disease or condition. Treatment plans are discussed with your physician. In fact, you may be in the midst of treatment. Decisions about the end of life are less abstract, becoming more relevant as you live with some decline to your health.

Stage Three: You are nearing the end of your life, likely within the next six to twelve months. Decisions about your end-of-life preferences are now real and urgent.

Planning can and should occur at *each* stage. The details of your preferences will likely change as you move from stage to stage. Remember that 90 percent of us will experience a decline in health over time. For most of us, moving through stages two and three will occur over months or years; we will have time to plan. Those who begin planning at stage one will be prepared to revisit and revise decisions in stage two. Similarly, those realistically addressing their condition in stage two will be prepared to revisit and revise their decisions as the end draws near.

If you are currently in stage two or three, I highly recommend advance care planning with a facilitator. Ask your physician if such services are available in your area. Investigate whether a local hospital has palliative care specialists who can assist you. If none are formally available, seek out a nurse, social worker, or other professional who can patiently guide you through a conversation about your choices.

Additionally, in stage two and three, you should ask for time with your physician to walk through the course of your disease and the possible outcomes that could lead to the end of your life. Chapter 10 provides a variety of questions and topics to include in this conversation.

When Intervention Is Required

In order to express your medical decisions, you must first understand the circumstances in which your directive would most likely be exercised if you were unable to make or communicate your own medical decisions. Not all circumstances can be anticipated. Nonetheless, healthcare directives typically reflect the following broad and significant circumstances when you could become unable to make or communicate your treatment preferences:

- **If you became terminally ill or terminally injured:** Your primary (or attending) doctor and another qualified doctor decide that you have an irreversible, incurable condition from which you will not recover.

- **If you were in a persistent vegetative state:** Your primary (or attending) doctor and another qualified doctor agree that, within a reasonable degree of medical certainty, you can no longer feel anything, knowingly move, or be aware of being alive. *You have been in this state for at least four weeks.* They are qualified to make this diagnosis, believe this condition will last indefinitely without hope for improvement, and have observed you long enough to make that decision.

- **If you became permanently unconscious:** Your primary (or attending) doctor and another qualified doctor agree that, within a reasonable degree of medical certainty, you can no longer feel anything, knowingly move, or be aware of being alive. *You have been in this state for at least one year.* They are qualified to make this diagnosis, believe this condition will last indefinitely without hope for improvement, and have observed you long enough to make that decision.

- **If you were suffering from advanced dementia:** Your primary (or attending) doctor and another qualified doctor agree that you have an irreversible brain injury or a progressive brain disease from which you will not recover, and that you have reached an advanced state of dementia or memory loss where you are permanently unable to communicate, recognize your loved ones, care for yourself, eat, and drink by yourself.

- **If you were dying from a progressive disease** such as Amyotrophic lateral sclerosis (A.L.S., also called Lou Gehrig's disease), Tays-Sachs, or some forms of multiple sclerosis (M.S.): Your primary (or attending) doctor and another qualified doctor agree that you have a progressive disease from which you will not recover, and that you have reached an advanced state where you are permanently unable to communicate, care for yourself, eat, and drink by yourself.

- **If you were extremely frail from aging, and have been admitted to the hospital for a common affliction or injury:** Death is not always triggered by disease. Our bodies can simply wear out. Through your healthcare directive, you can exercise your right to limit or refuse treatment in this circumstance.

• **If you were temporarily incapacitated from an accident or sudden medical event:** Though healthcare directives are most commonly applicable for end-of-life care, a directive can be immensely helpful to your medical team and your healthcare agent if you should temporarily lose the ability to make or communicate your own decisions.

Level of Intervention

In any of those circumstances, the fundamental question is the level of intervention, or care, you wish to receive. Imagine if you could speak for yourself in that moment, which of the following three choices would you pick?

1. Request all life-sustaining treatment in an effort to extend your life as long as possible. Life-sustaining treatment includes medical treatments, interventions, and procedures that keep a patient alive by taking over or restoring vital bodily function(s).[30] Some treatments address what is medically urgent (acute), such as cardiopulmonary resuscitation (C.P.R.) to keep your heart beating and to ensure you are breathing, which might require mechanical assistance by placing you on a ventilator. Life-sustaining treatment also includes measures to enable you to continue living—that sustain you—such as kidney dialysis, surgery, artificially administered nutrition (food) and hydration (fluids), blood transfusions, administration of antibiotics and other drugs, and other medical procedures.[31] In medical terminology, this is also referred to as "Full Code" and "Full Support."

Many people deeply value the sanctity of life. Regardless of the potential suffering or pain, some individuals hold that all possible medical care should be delivered in every circumstance, believing in the possibility of recovery, and that they will beat the odds. Others fear death and prefer to risk negative consequences to extend life as long as possible. If any of these statements reflect your view, be sure to state your wish to receive all life-sustaining treatment in your healthcare directive.

Even if you request all possible care, your physician can choose to limit the treatments used according to what he deems medically appropriate. For example, an emergency physician could refuse to administer C.P.R. on a frail ninety-seven-year-old patient who is actively dying, or a patient with extremely advanced terminal cancer.

2. Request to Allow a Natural Death, abbreviated as A.N.D. This is a relatively new medical term, intended to replace "Do Not Resuscitate" or D.N.R. as well as ambiguous phrases such as "no heroic measures" or "I don't want to be hooked up to machines."

Ruth Wittman-Price, nursing department chair at Francis Marion University, South Carolina, explains: "The phrase 'Do Not Resuscitate' signals an intent to withhold or refuse. It says you're not going to do something. To 'Allow Natural Death,' on the other hand, connotes permission."[32] The tone of permission enables loved ones to more readily accept the dying process. Though not adopted universally, the phrase "Allow Natural Death" is catching on and is embraced by most hospitals.

As the name suggests, A.N.D. shifts the emphasis from pursuing curative treatment or treatment that would interfere with the dying process, to administering comfort care. It is far broader than D.N.R., as it includes more procedures. A.N.D. includes:

- *Do not* resuscitate (also referred to as "No Code").

- *Do not* intubate (ventilate; also considered part of "No Code").

- *Do not* administer antibiotics or curative medications.

- *Do not* administer artificial nutrition (food) or hydration (fluids).

- *Do not* perform kidney dialysis.

- *Do not* interfere with the natural dying process.

- *Do not* admit to hospital, unless only addressing symptoms and comfort care.

- *Do* provide comfort care (note the positive statement). It is important to emphasize that you can still request and should receive comfort care measures even if you want to allow a natural death. More about comfort care is discussed later in this chapter.

3. Limit the type of care you receive. You may establish guidelines for limiting your care. It is nearly impossible to anticipate the types of treatments your medical team could recommend. Therefore, consider expressing limits through generalized statements that could guide decisions and be applied in multiple medical circumstances.

> *Time:* You can request that you receive treatment for a trial period only. That may make it easier for your loved ones and medical team to withdraw treatment if you are not responding.

> > *For example:* Being willing to be placed on a ventilator for a trial period (days or weeks) in an effort to give your body time to recover from pneumonia, yet being unwilling to remain on a ventilator for months.

> *Type of condition:* You can ask to receive treatment only for a reversible condition. A few examples include: skin infection, bladder infection, bronchitis, uncom-

plicated pneumonia, bacterial pharyngitis, bacterial sinusitis, uncomplicated eye infection (pink eye).

> *For example:* Receiving antibiotics for several days in an effort to address a bladder infection, even when diagnosed with terminal cancer and requesting no resuscitation.

Purpose for treatment: You can state that treatment should be directed at prolonging a meaningful quality of life, as you have defined it, versus prolonging the dying process.

> *For example:* Accepting dialysis while you are still able to recognize loved ones in spite of dementia, yet choosing to have treatment withheld or withdrawn if you can no longer recognize those you hold dear.

Exclusions: You may specify any number of exclusions.

> *For example:* Common exclusions include C.P.R., intubation (ventilation), dialysis, antibiotics for life-threatening infection (such as pneumonia), electroconvulsive therapy, psychotropic drugs, pregnancy termination, sterilization, amputation of any limbs, blood transfusion for religious reasons, and more. Speak with your doctor about what exclusions are appropriate to meet your preferences and personal beliefs for end-of-life care.

Alternatives: You can specify alternative treatments.

> *For example:* You could state that you do not want tubes put in your nose or throat for breathing, but that you are willing to receive external breathing assistance, with a tightly fitting oxygen

mask. This is called "positive airway pressure." Or, you can state a preference for alternative pain management, such as acupuncture or other non-traditional therapies.

Previously, I mentioned that studies show the majority of individuals would prefer a natural death, rather than invasive treatment at the end of life. In fact, many of the states' directive forms are based on the right to refuse care.

The majority of patients or healthcare agents making the decision for the patient choose the middle road. Minimally, most want to receive comfort-care measures while avoiding invasive treatments. Those with dementia may opt out of treatments that could restore them physically, preferring death to the ongoing loss of memory over time.

Be judicious about healthcare instructions that are exceedingly restrictive, allowing no care. Similarly, be cautious about requesting all possible care if you have any concerns about being hooked up to machines for months or even years, if that should be required. Like most, you could opt to limit your care. Describing the middle road requires careful consideration. A conversation with your physician is strongly advised to help you articulate what is right for you.

Talk with your healthcare provider about the level of intervention that is right for you:

- All life-sustaining treatment
- Allow natural death
- Limited treatment

Artificially Administered Nutrition and Hydration

The Terri Schiavo case (referenced in chapter 4) highlighted the implications of artificially administering nutrition (food) and hydration (fluids) to sustain life over many years. Many state statutes now require the principal to expressly indicate her desire to receive artificially administered food and fluids indefinitely or to have it withheld or withdrawn if the patient will not recover. Food and fluids are artificially administered by a tube that is inserted through the stomach wall, nose, mouth, or into a vein. It is important to note that the term "artificially administered feeding" does not include non-intrusive methods of feeding, such as spoon feeding a patient or moistening a patient's lips for comfort. Additionally, some amount of artificial fluids may be required to administer some types of comfort medication.

Inserting a feeding tube is considered routine by many hospitals and nursing homes, often without fully discussing the implications with the patient or loved ones. It is frequently administered in older patients and those with dementia. One study reported the following:

- "Nearly 14 percent of those with a relative who had a feeding tube inserted reported that there was 'no discussion with a healthcare provider' prior to the procedure.

- Another 10 percent said that they felt pressured by the physician to put in a feeding tube.

- More than 30 percent reported that they were not informed of the risks of tube insertion.

- Nearly 40 percent said the tube bothered their relative.

- In addition, 33 percent of those with a feeding tube were reported to be physically or pharmacologically restrained."[33]

Even if a patient clearly will not recover, often families struggle with the morality of removing artificially administered food and fluids. If your directive states that you want to receive food and fluids, be clear whether you expect this to continue indefinitely. Alternatively, consider defining a period of time after which, if you are not recovering, the tubes should be removed. Make this decision easier for your loved ones by proactively defining how long you wish to receive artificially administered food and fluids.

Consider the degree to which you would be willing to be restrained in order to have food and water artificially administered. Also decide if you would limit the duration if you are not recovering. Express your wishes clearly in your directive.

Comfort Care (Palliative Care)

Perhaps the greatest anxiety we feel regarding the end of life is the fear of pain and suffering during the dying process. Thankfully, medical practices in our country have made significant progress in the past decade in delivering comfort care, also known as palliative care. Most major hospitals have incorporated the specialty of palliative care. Your healthcare directive can include specific instructions for your comfort care.

Comfort care is defined as care that focuses on managing symptoms, pain, and discomfort. Comfort care does not aim to cure the disease or condition, but rather to reduce and alleviate any suffering in order to improve the patient's quality of life.

A wide range of medications can manage pain, nausea, and other symptoms in order to promote the best possible quality of life. In fact, comfort care can truly optimize quality of life for patients with progressive illness. Suffering need not occur. Comfort care can be administered at **any time** during the management of a disease; it is not limited to the final days as a patient approaches death. Furthermore, multiple methods are available to administer pain medication: orally, via a patch, through an I.V. or a shot, a spray, or a pill placed under the tongue or in the rectum. In other words, even if you cannot swallow, or do not want an I.V. or a shot, you can successfully receive pain medication.

Comfort care can be administered to varying degrees, based upon balancing three objectives. These comfort care goals are **not** mutually exclusive. Rather, the art of comfort care lies in balancing the interdependence of these three goals according to your wishes. The goals are:

Comfort: Managing pain and discomfort and controlling symptoms to reduce and even eliminate suffering.

Function: Allowing for the greatest level of functioning, including thinking, communication, and movement.

Longevity: Extending life as long as possible.

The following stories show the interdependence of these goals.

George is an elderly man with Parkinson's disease who is also experiencing significant joint pain. George might prefer to **strongly manage his pain and symptoms,** however this will reduce his ability to communicate and interact with his loved ones. He acknowledges that the pain medication may hasten his death. George's highest priority is comfort, then function; longevity is least important.

Kim is a mid-sixties mother with congestive heart failure. Her daughter's wedding is just two months away. Kim has been having more frequent episodes with breathing difficulty. The most recent landed her in the emergency room. Kim may wish to **preserve her functional ability** above all in order to participate in planning the final details and then attending her daughter's wedding. She chooses to limit her symptom medications in order to maintain her mental focus. Her highest priorities are function and longevity, which may require compromising her level of comfort.

Steve is a young father with end-stage cancer. He may **choose longevity as his highest priority.** He chooses to moderate his pain medication; he primarily manages his discomfort through meditation and homeopathic remedies in order to minimize the impact to his functional ability. His hope is to spend as much time as possible with his two young children and his wife, giving them good memories of their time together. Longevity and function are Steve's highest priorities.

Decisions on the priorities for comfort care can vary, based on the circumstances of your life. This is yet another reason to refresh your healthcare directive every few years. Also, it is vital to have a healthcare agent who will strongly advocate for your comfort.

Given your present state of health, how would you prioritize your goals for comfort care?
- Comfort
- Longevity
- Function

Suffering is NOT a given at the end of life.
Include your comfort care priorities in your healthcare directive.

Secondary Decisions

The value of hospice care

Hospice care can be an amazing gift to dying patients and their loved ones. Hospice emphasizes comfort care instead of curative care. It attends to the emotional, social, and spiritual needs of patients and their loved ones as they journey through the dying process. For those who have walked this path with someone, the most common observation is "we should have moved our loved one to hospice sooner."

Some people may be confused regarding the distinction between comfort care and hospice. The primary purpose of hospice care is the provision of humane and compassionate medical, emotional, and spiritual care to the dying patient—as well as their loved ones. Hospice focuses on the patient's quality—not length—of life, offering comfort care to effectively manage pain and other symptoms. Additionally, hospice recognizes and honors the role of loved ones in the dying process. By caring for the family as well as the patient, hospice enables loved ones to focus on living and loving. Many hospice organizations also offer bereavement support for loved ones.

Hospice is a style of care, not a physical location. It can be delivered in several settings, including home, nursing homes, hospitals, or specialized hospice facilities. Patients can receive hospice care for days, weeks, or even months. Although many hospice patients have a diagnosis of cancer, patients with any end-stage condition can, and do, receive hospice care. Individuals with advanced illnesses such as heart disease, lung disease, Alzheimer's disease or dementia, stroke, or kidney failure can also choose hospice services. Hospice care is covered by most private insurance carriers and Medicare.

Some hospitals are proactive, offering hospice to a patient who has a terminal illness. Both longevity and quality of life often improve in hospice care, as a patient shifts his focus to experiencing life and love as long as possible, in lieu of enduring difficult treatments, such as chemotherapy. In fact, research published in the *Journal of Pain and Symptom Management* found that terminally ill patients who received hospice care lived on average twenty-nine days longer than those who did not opt for hospice near the end of life.[34]

Some hospitals or physicians are not prepared to introduce the concept of hospice care, worrying that it signals surrender and will discourage their patient. Likewise, loved ones may be reluctant to suggest hospice for fear it indicates an unwillingness to support a patient's effort to beat a disease. You can spare your loved ones from the difficulty of wondering whether or not to suggest hospice by including your instructions to pursue hospice for end-of-life care in your healthcare directive.

When symptoms and pain are effectively managed, and

emotional and spiritual needs are attended to, patients in a hospice setting can pass peacefully, with dignity, surrounded by loved ones. Notably, those well cared for in hospice rarely ask for euthanasia or physician-assisted suicide.

Medicare pays for most hospice care in the United States. To receive Medicare hospice benefits, the patient must be eligible for Medicare Part A and receive care from a Medicare-approved hospice program. Importantly, Medicare requires a physician to document a prognosis that the patient has fewer than six months to live. Arriving at a precise timeline is difficult to achieve, and many physicians are unwilling or uncomfortable projecting how long a patient will live. Additionally, the patient must sign a statement that he or she is choosing hospice care instead of other Medicare-covered benefits to treat terminal illness. Medicare will still pay for covered benefits according to its standard practices for any health problems that aren't related to the terminal illness. Any patient can stop hospice and return to pursuing curative care at any time. Finally, if hospice is required beyond the sixth month, the medical team can re-certify the patient for another benefit period.

Hospice care improves the quality of end of life for most individuals. It allows the patient to experience life and love as long as possible rather than endure difficult treatments when a cure or recovery is no longer possible. Consider your preference and include your choice regarding hospice in your directive.

Organ Donation

Did you know that nineteen people in the U.S. die each day waiting for an organ transplant? Organ donation can be a surprising comfort to families struggling to make sense over the loss of a loved one, particularly when the death occurs suddenly and unexpectedly. However, families may hesitate, for lack of knowing your wishes.

> One-third of consenting donors never realize their wish to donate because family members subsequently refuse permission—in many cases simply because they are unaware of their loved one's preference.

If you desire to donate your organs and tissue, empower your healthcare agent in your directive to authorize this life-saving gift. You can choose to donate all, or only part of, your organs and tissue. For example, a woman friend does not want her eyes removed. A business colleague whose internal organs were damaged by disease donated his skin to help burn victims. You can even define the purpose for your donation: therapy or treatment (organ transplant), research (studying an organ to understand the disease), or education (used for teaching medical students).

The recipient's health insurance covers the cost. The donating family does not bear the financial burden of the transplant, nor do they receive any payment for the organ or tissue.

One of the unexpected stresses families experience as they are coping with a loss is the need to answer numerous social and medical questions about their loved one as part of the organ donation process. This can be overwhelming and certainly feel intrusive. Consider registering in advance as an organ donor. You can answer all of the questions in advance, removing this burden from your loved ones. Contact your local hospital, or speak with your physician, to learn which registry provides service in your area. Check the *Resources* section for additional information about organ donation registration.

If you are including organ donation in your directive, consider taking the time to have this designation added to your driver's license. It is important to note that if a discrepancy exists between your driver's license organ donor designation and your healthcare directive, whichever was most recently written and executed will prevail.

Autopsy

Consider whether you would empower your healthcare agent to authorize an autopsy that could explain the cause of your death to your loved ones. Alternatively, an autopsy could be authorized to advance medical science. For example, our family chose to donate my mother's brain to the Mayo Clinic's Alzheimer's research study. Be advised that a judge, sheriff, or medical examiner can order an autopsy, if warranted, against your wishes.

Other Considerations

Finally, your healthcare directive could possibly include other considerations, such as your desire to participate in a clinical trial, your wishes if you were pregnant (should the fetus be brought to term), and where you would prefer to die (home, hospital or somewhere else).

Providers and Insurance

Including your preferred doctors and hospitals can be invaluable to your healthcare agent and loved ones. If you have more than one residence, include information for multiple locations. Additionally, include your insurance information, and where you keep your insurance card(s).

Financial Boundaries

Some individuals prefer to establish financial limits for their end-of-life health care. This topic is deeply private for many individuals, and therefore, difficult to discuss. If you want the financial implications of your treatment choices to be a factor in the decision-making process, make this point clearly in your healthcare directive. Provide specific instructions instead of vague statements.

Consider, as well, whether you would accept a financial gift from a loved one for your care if your assets do not cover the expenses. Adult children sometimes intervene in the care for their aging parent, stating, "I'll pay for all of this. Just save Mom." However, Mom may have already reached the decision to allow a natural death. Whether motivated by love or guilt, the adult child can push for more treatment by addressing a financial gap. Other family members could yield under duress. Make your boundaries clear as part of your directive.

P.O.L.S.T. and D.N.R. Forms

Physician Orders for Life-Sustaining Treatment

In recent years, many states have adopted a new type of end-of-life document called a P.O.L.S.T. This document goes by multiple names (see the list included in chapter 3). The P.O.L.S.T. is a one-to-two-page form and is typically printed on a bright-colored piece of paper, such as orange or hot pink.

The P.O.L.S.T. communicates the doctor's orders regarding a patient's goals for care: receive all possible treatment, limited treatment, or allow a natural death. It includes instructions regarding:

- Attempting resuscitation (C.P.R.),

- Pursuing intubation (ventilation),

- Administering antibiotics,

- Administering artificial food and hydration,

- Pursuing aggressive curative treatment,

- Transferring the patient to the emergency room,

- Admitting the patient to the hospital (versus managing comfort care at the residence),

- Balancing the goals for comfort care: comfort, function and longevity,

- Emphasizing dignity and respect for the patient.

The P.O.L.S.T. is not necessary for everyone. It is a supplement for a healthcare directive, not a substitute. It is intended for those who are nearing the end whose death might occur in the next six to twelve months. While a P.O.L.S.T. can be written to pursue aggressive treatment intended to cure the underlying condition, most P.O.L.S.T. documents are written to limit treatment and emphasize comfort care.

Because the P.O.L.S.T. document is written as a doctor's orders, all medical personnel, including E.M.T.s, are required to follow its instructions. A healthcare directive is not a doctor's order. This is a critical distinction.

Many families experience tremendous frustration and confusion when a healthcare directive is presented to the

E.M.T.s in an emergency, yet in spite of the instructions to give comfort care only, the E.M.T.s will administer all possible care to revive and stabilize the patient. In many jurisdictions, E.M.T.s are required to do just that: They must perform C.P.R. and/or intubate the patient, even if a healthcare directive indicates a patient's choice to allow a natural death. This is a limitation of a healthcare directive and is one of the reasons for the invention of the P.O.L.S.T.

The P.O.L.S.T. document is intended to move with the patient through his care, whether at home, in the ambulance, at a hospital emergency room, as an admitted hospital patient, or in a nursing home or hospice facility. It should be easily retrievable by those who need it. Chapter 10 provides specific instructions on storing and posting your P.O.L.S.T.

The P.O.L.S.T. simplifies and strengthens how your medical wishes are communicated to your medical team. Speak with your physician about writing a P.O.L.S.T. with, and for, you. States have different forms, and even hospitals can have a form preference, so start with your physician.

While the P.O.L.S.T. serves a valuable function and has been embraced by the medical community, the legal community has voiced reasonable concern. While some states require the signature of the patient to whom the P.O.L.S.T. applies, others do not. In those states, a P.O.L.S.T. can be created for a patient, based on a conversation between the attending physician and loved ones, in the absence of a healthcare directive or legally assigned healthcare agent. When the patient has not expressed his wishes through a legal healthcare directive, loved ones may seek to minimize suffering by requesting that the physician allow a natural death. That may be a loving act. Unfortunately, someone with a sinister objective can also be motivated to make the same request. It may be impossible for a physician to discern whether family members are seeking a P.O.L.S.T. to avoid suffering and a prolonged death for their loved one or to accelerate the death of someone for financial or selfish motives.

If you are elderly, struggling with complex medical issues, or if you have been diagnosed with a life-limiting illness, a P.O.L.S.T. is highly recommended in addition to your healthcare directive.

Completing a Do Not Resuscitate (D.N.R) or Allow Natural Death (A.N.D.) Order

In some states and hospitals, the P.O.L.S.T. has replaced the D.N.R. form. However, in other states and hospitals, the D.N.R. form remains, and some states use both. In some cases, a physician simply notes D.N.R. on the patient's chart. Nurses often note D.N.R. on a patient's whiteboard in the room.

As it denotes, the D.N.R. order communicates to your medical team that you do not want to receive C.P.R. or ventilation or drugs used in an attempt to restart your heart or breathing. Though the phrase is "Do Not Resuscitate," it generally includes "Do Not Intubate" as well. Like the P.O.L.S.T., it must be authorized by a physician. Medical teams use the phrase "No Code" to describe a patient who does not want to be resuscitated.

More and more hospitals have adopted the phrase "Allow Natural Death (A.N.D.)" because the word **not** in "Do Not Resuscitate" causes fear and confusion for both patients and families. Though a D.N.R. is not meant to signify do not treat, just the possibility raises concern.

Out-of-Hospital D.N.R.

Some states require a separate form to ensure your wishes for allowing a natural death or D.N.R. are followed by those outside of the hospital. This includes emergency, nursing home, or assisted-living personnel. In many states, the P.O.L.S.T. has replaced this form. In some states, a separate "Home Do Not Resuscitate" form may be required.

Addressing Possible Document Confusion

Several differences by state, and the evolution of end-of-life documentation, leave us with multiple forms and options. As stated in chapter 3, the lack of a national standard leaves room for confusion. The information presented could seem overwhelming. Re-read this chapter when the time seems right. To clarify:

- Every adult should write a healthcare directive. Chapter 5 addresses three possible scenarios to guide you; choose what is right for you.

- Individuals with a terminal or chronic disease, and the elderly, will benefit from additional forms that explain your wishes as a doctor's order in a P.O.L.S.T. and/or D.N.R. to anyone who delivers medical care.

If you are uncertain on how to proceed, schedule a meeting with your physician to discuss which form(s) are appropriate for your circumstance and applicable in your state. Be certain all forms written are in agreement and communicate your wishes consistently.

Situational Directives

Prior to any form of surgery or medical procedure, review your directive and assess whether you would be best served to create a brief, separate document that explains your instructions specific to this surgery. Physicians often ask, "If anything happens during the surgery and your heart stops, what do you want us to do?" While you may choose to allow a natural death in the case of a terminal illness, you could feel just the opposite in the case of surgery. If your heart stopped during surgery, you could state your instructions to receive C.P.R. and all measures to restart your heart and breathing.

In Summary

This chapter has highlighted difficult and sobering choices and the necessity to record specific preferences. Writing your healthcare instructions requires many significant decisions:

- Determining the level of intervention you want to receive,
- Choosing whether to receive artificially administered food and fluids,
- Defining your goals for comfort care,
- Expressing your interest in hospice care,
- Authorizing organ donation or an autopsy,
- Establishing financial limits for your care,
- Determining whether a P.O.L.S.T. or D.N.R. is appropriate for your circumstance and, if so, completing the form(s) with your physician.

These decisions are critical to express your specific wishes for the end of your life. Every one of us will die. While denial seems convenient in the short term, the long term requires your attention so your family is better prepared if (or when) faced with a crisis situation. When you write out and clearly express your healthcare directive, you give your loved ones a gift only you can give. You also give yourself peace of mind.

8

How to Select a Healthcare Agent Who Will Advocate for Your Wishes

Who will advocate for your preferences if you are unable to speak for yourself? It is very important that you choose your healthcare agent carefully and thoughtfully.

What Is the Role of a Healthcare Agent?

A healthcare agent is the person you authorize to make treatment decisions on your behalf if you are unable to communicate or are mentally unable to make your own decisions. Generally, the role includes the authority to allow, refuse, or withdraw your medical treatments. A healthcare agent has legal power of attorney, but only for medical decisions. The role of healthcare agent does *not* include the authority to handle medical expenses or financial transactions related to your treatment. For this and other financial needs, a financial power of attorney is required. You can select the same person to serve both as healthcare agent and as

As a reminder, when terms were introduced in chapter 3, I noted that the term healthcare agent in the singular form is used in this book for the sake of simplicity. However, I strongly urge you to select at least one, if not two, alternate agents. Therefore, the recommendations that are offered in this chapter will mostly likely apply to two or three people.

your financial power of attorney or choose separate people for these important roles. See *Financial Management* later in this chapter for further explanation.

Your healthcare agent serves as your advocate, pursuing your treatment preferences when you are unable to do so. In practical terms, this means your healthcare agent is the person who meets with the medical team to discuss possible treatment choices. Based upon your healthcare instructions (see chapter 7), your agent will choose which treatments to pursue or withhold. Your agent could even be required to instruct your physician to withdraw treatment that is only prolonging your dying or that is causing suffering without the hope of recovery. Your agent can ask for a second opinion, seek out care from a specialist, or request your transfer to another hospital if any of these actions best serve your interests according to your directive. Some states allow a healthcare agent to request an autopsy and/or to donate your organs and tissue after your death. Your agent could also facilitate the transfer of your remains to a mortuary after you have died.

> Your chosen healthcare agent is **your voice,** advocating for your healthcare treatment choices when you are unable to make or communicate your own preferences.

Additionally, your healthcare agent might have to navigate through the difficult and painful emotions of those surrounding you at the end of your life. Some loved ones who do not agree with your stated preferences might challenge your agent's decisions on your behalf. Your agent may have to act as a facilitator to help your family unite and accept your chosen treatment wishes.

Having One Primary versus Multiple Agents

Most attorneys and advisors recommend choosing one individual as your primary healthcare agent. Having a primary agent will prevent contradictory decisions made by multiple agents who are unable to agree during a stressful time.

It is critical to select one or more alternate agents. In case your primary agent is unavailable or unable to serve in this role when needed, an alternate can be called upon. Most forms or tools highly recommend that you select at least one alternate. It is worth noting that, in most states, if the spouse was named as the primary agent—and a divorce or annulment occurs—that role is revoked and the alternate agent will be engaged as the decision-maker.

Some individuals might decide to have two or more loved ones share the decision-making. Family dynamics can make it difficult to select one agent. Or, some might feel that two or three loved ones can better carry the weight of the decision together. In this case, it is important to identify who will have *final* authority if consensus is not reached. In a situation where agents with equal authority disagree about decisions concerning the patient's care, the decision is typically referred to an ethics committee at the treating hospital. Ethics committees are positioned to respond promptly in most hospitals.

Selecting Your Healthcare Agent and Alternates

Choose agents you *trust*, who know you well, and who are strong. Choose agents who will:

- Advocate strongly for *your preferences,* even if it requires setting aside their own wishes or beliefs.

- Hold firm to your directive and not be swayed by well-meaning loved ones who earnestly believe a different treatment decision would serve you best.

- Assertively, even aggressively, engage the medical team in providing the best possible care for you, as you've defined it. This could include diagnostics, disease treatment, and/or comfort care. If required, it could include pursuing a transfer to another hospital. Choose someone who can go toe-to-toe with medical or hospital professionals if it becomes necessary.

- Passionately assert your need for comfort care, since some hospitals are not staffed with palliative care specialists.

- Be trusted by your extended family.

- Remain strong through the course of difficult emotions and stress.

- Take time to learn the medical details of your situation, and seek medical advice when it is warranted. Selecting an agent with medical knowledge is beneficial, if someone in your circle of loved ones also meets the other above criteria. A healthcare agent who understands the course of your disease will be more discerning about whether a transfer to an emergency room or the hospital is necessary.

Selecting your healthcare agent and alternates is perhaps the most important decision of the entire healthcare directive. Choose wisely.

Get Permission from Your Agent and Alternates

Talk with your healthcare agent and alternates to ensure those you choose are willing and able to make medical decisions for you, as some of the decisions could be difficult. It is critical that your chosen healthcare agents understand and accept this role. You might learn that someone you would like to appoint is unwilling or feels unable to serve in this capacity. Better to find out now, respect that decision, and choose someone else. It can be helpful to explain that your agents' personal finances are not at risk by agreeing to serve in this role. Additionally, as a means of supporting your agents, your directive can include a provision to hire or engage a care manager if your medical treatment becomes complex.

About the Authority You Are Giving

The role of a healthcare agent, as described above, explains what functions an agent typically performs. However, you can, and should, specify the authority you are giving to your agent. You can make a broad statement such as, "My healthcare agent has the power to make decisions that are in my best interest." This statement is vague, so be cautious. If you have written clear healthcare instructions, a sweeping best-interest approach may work for you. Alternatively, you can spell out individual points of authority, such as having the authority for:

- Making decisions to give, refuse, or withdraw any treatment or procedure.

- Choosing who provides your health care, including both the individuals and/or the hospitals.

- Deciding where you live and receive care, including other states, if your location relates to your health care.

- Having access to your medical records. Your healthcare directive should include language that authorizes a medical facility to release your information under HIPAA rules.

- Dealing with any other decisions you choose.

Set Limitations

Generally speaking, your healthcare agent's authority is limited by your healthcare instructions. Some people wish to restrict the authority of their agent by setting specific limitations, stating, "My healthcare agent cannot authorize:"

- electroshock therapy
- administering psychotropic drugs
- pregnancy termination
- sterilization
- admission to a mental institution
- assisted suicide
- euthanasia
- anything else you choose

Who Cannot Be Your Healthcare Agent

Some people are not allowed to serve as your healthcare agent. Because the rules differ by state, be certain to check your state's statutes. Most states have laws in place to protect a patient by placing limits on who can serve as an agent. The limits are intended to prevent any actual or perceived conflict of interest. In general, you **cannot** choose a person who:

- Is younger than eighteen years of age (nineteen in some states).

- Requests to be named your healthcare agent as a condition of:

  - Your admission to a healthcare facility, community-care facility, or residential-care facility,

  - Treatment you receive.

- Is directly or indirectly responsible for providing your health care. This includes your healthcare providers or their spouses, employees of your healthcare provider or their spouses, or the operators, owners, administrators or employees of a healthcare facility, a community-care facility, or a residential-care facility where you are receiving care unless they are related to you by blood, marriage or adoption.

A few states also stipulate that your healthcare agent cannot be:

- An employee of a government agency that is financially responsible for your care, or

- Any person serving as an agent for ten or more persons.

What Happens When You Have Not Named an Agent?

If you should become unable to make or communicate your own healthcare decisions, and have not named a healthcare agent, those decisions can be made by a myriad of possible people. Rules differ by state. The spouse is most commonly recognized as the first in priority to make end-of-life decisions. However, as the Terri Schiavo case demonstrated, a spouse is not necessarily the final voice. In most states, the spouse is followed by adult children, parents, and siblings, in that order. In some states, the attending physician selects the decision-maker from those who are available, based on whomever they believe will make the best decisions for the patient. Of course, the physician would likely choose someone who agrees with his point of view. In some states, decision-making is left to the attending physician after consulting with the family. In certain circumstances, a court can name a guardian or conservator.

It is highly unlikely that your end-of-life decisions will make national news or be prolonged for multiple years. Nonetheless, this is a great example of the need to be prepared. That's why it's called *advance* care planning.

> A decision-maker will be chosen if you are unable to speak for yourself. It is much better for you to make that choice in advance.

Guardian Versus Healthcare Agent

You have the ability to choose a healthcare agent, but if you do not, and if decisions are required for your property or for your health care, a court can choose a guardian. A guardian has the authority to make healthcare decisions on your behalf **and** to manage your property and financial matters. A healthcare agent has the authority only to make healthcare decisions. To ensure that your wishes are followed by a person that you trust, select a healthcare agent and make the selection legal through a health-care power of attorney as part of your healthcare directive.

Protect Yourself From the Wrong Decision-Maker

In some families, it can be equally important to record in writing those who should **not** participate in making healthcare decisions on your behalf. Families are complicated. Heightened emotions in a crisis can stir up old wounds. Be proactive and protect yourself from the wrong decision-maker. It might be a sibling who believes all possible treatment should be pursued, and you prefer to allow a natural death. Or, it might just be that your spouse or one of your children would struggle mightily if a time comes when your family needs to let you go. Consider protecting him or her from participating in the painful decision to pull the plug, while protecting you from unwanted treatment that prolongs the dying process.

Financial Management

As mentioned previously, a healthcare power of attorney document gives the authority to your healthcare agent to make **only** medical decisions. A separate document, called a Financial Power of Attorney, is required to empower an individual to make financial decisions and execute financial transactions on your behalf. You can select the same person to serve in both roles, but two separate documents are required. While a spouse might be able to execute financial decisions, circumstances can be complex and are certainly unique to individuals and to each situation.

> Consult with an attorney to determine if you should complete a financial power of attorney document. Additionally, seek the counsel of an attorney and/or your accountant for estate planning advice.

Legal Protection

The person you ask to serve as your healthcare agent has a formidable responsibility. Typically two provisions are designed to protect healthcare agents:

1. Your healthcare agent does not incur any liability for the decisions made.

2. Your healthcare agent is given the same constitutional rights as you would have, if you were making your own decisions.

Challenging Your Chosen Healthcare Agent

If a healthcare agent is not willing or able to make decisions that align with the principal's healthcare instructions, it is possible to challenge the principal's chosen healthcare agent, and have him removed. For example, I could name my husband as my agent. My instructions could clearly state that I do not want to be placed on a ventilator for more than two weeks. If my husband was unwilling to pull the plug after this trial period, my brother could challenge the appointment through the hospital ethics committee, or, if necessary, in court. My brother could ask to become my guardian. That takes time, money to pay the attorneys, and adds pain and aggravation for me, my husband, my brother, and other loved ones. This is even more reason to choose wisely.

In Summary

Thoughtful selection of your healthcare agent and alternates is crucial. It is a difficult job and a solemn responsibility. Conversation is required. Ask your agents if they are willing to accept this role. They should not be blind-sided. Your agents should have the liberty to ask questions and discuss your wishes until each is confident in his understanding of your preferences. If your chosen agent and alternates clearly understand your choices and are committed to advocating on your behalf, you have the strongest likelihood of having your wishes honored.

9

Support Your Loved Ones
So They Can Fully Support You

How your life ends will deeply affect those you love. Remember, this is not just about you. If your death occurs suddenly, loved ones might be unprepared. Alternatively, if you experience a slow decline, loved ones will struggle with you through the dying process. Ultimately, they will want to honor and celebrate your life.

While your medical instructions and your choice of healthcare agent are the legal core of your document, exploring the emotional, social, financial, and spiritual dimensions at the end of life are vital for you and for your loved ones. Through your written healthcare directive, you have the opportunity to express important messages to those you hold dear. You can provide guidance to help your loved ones understand concrete ways to support you through the dying process. Finally, you can convey your hopes for how your life can be celebrated.

Messages to Loved Ones

If you knew a loved one—perhaps an aging parent—had forty-eight hours to live, would you strive to resolve any unfinished emotional business before their passing? Are there words you hope you could hear or say one more time— perhaps, "I love you?"

If you knew you had only a matter of days to live:

- What messages could you share with your loved ones that would provide comfort?

- Would you strive to mend any relationships?

- Are there words that need to be said?

In his book *The Four Things That Matter Most*,[35] Dr. Ira Byock shares four key phrases that can help families through difficult and challenging circumstances: "Please forgive me," "I forgive you," "Thank you," and "I love you." Each of us has the opportunity to share these phrases with our loved ones throughout our lives. They can also be particularly comforting to those loved ones who are making difficult decisions on our behalf. Communicating such messages to loved ones is an important part of writing a comprehensive healthcare directive.

Personal Care

When a loved one is dying, we all want to *do* something. "Is there anything I can do?" is frequently asked by loved ones and friends who genuinely want to concretely express their love through action.

Your loved ones will be so grateful to have your wishes defined through your healthcare directive. For example, in the final weeks, days, or hours of your life:

- Would you like to have music playing in your room? What kind of music?

- Would you like to be read to? Are there favorite books or passages you would want to hear?

- Would you like lots of visitors? Just a few?

- Would you like your faith community to pray for you? A visit from a priest, pastor, rabbi or chaplain?

- Would you like to be shaved regularly if you are a man? Facial hair trimmed if you are an older woman?

- If you are easily chilled, would you like to be kept warm with extra blankets?

- Do you have seasonal allergies that require medication?

- Do you want to ask loved ones to care for a beloved pet?

As part of your healthcare directive, take the opportunity to express your needs for personal physical care (hygiene), emotional support, and spiritual support.

Cultural Diversity

Many hospitals have minimal, or no, training in the cultural norms regarding end-of-life conversation and expectations. Just as there is diversity in our society, there is diversity in how families from various ethnicities or faith traditions approach the dying process. Your medical team could be unprepared to address expectations specific to your heritage, whether those expectations emanate from faith-based practices, ethnicity, or even family-specific norms. For example, in some cultures, speaking openly about the dying process is considered forbidden. Assist your medical team and your healthcare agent by writing down, as part of your healthcare directive, any requirements or desires you have regarding your cultural practices at the end of your life.

Celebrating Your Life

One challenge that most adults face at some point in life is planning how best to honor the life of a loved one who has passed away. Families wrestle with many practical, as well as some very personal decisions, such as:

- Choosing a funeral home,

- Deciding whether a loved one will be buried or cremated,

- Deciding what clothes are suitable, if their loved one is to be buried,

- Determining whether to plan a visitation, open or closed casket, traditional funeral, memorial service, and/or graveside service to honor their loved one,

- Writing an obituary,

- Arranging for military honors for a veteran.

Your healthcare directive can ease the wondering and the work. Make your preferences known. Most families face these decisions at their worst time, when bereaved and vulnerable. In fact, a tremendous act of kindness towards your loved ones is to make your burial arrangements in advance, including the financial aspect. Check the *Resources* section for additional information.

Taking the time to explain how you want your life to be celebrated can lift the weight of these decisions from the shoulders of those you love most during a very difficult time.

Putting Your Affairs in Order

Writing your healthcare directive can serve as the impetus to put your worldly affairs in order. Have you written a will? If not, perhaps now is the time. If you have a will, does a trusted loved one know how to contact your attorney, or where to locate the document? What about other important papers such as a life insurance policy, deed to a home, or other documents? Do you have any personal items that you want to pass to certain children, grandchildren, nieces or nephews? If so, are these instructions written down and does anyone have a copy or know where to find a copy? Are there priceless family pictures stored in your home that you want to be sure are found and preserved? Do you have any cash or valuable jewelry hidden in books or other locations in your home? If so, does anyone know to retrieve these items after you have died, particularly if you live alone?

In today's on-line society, one often-overlooked aspect of preparation is providing appropriate access to passwords and login or user ID credentials for on-line accounts. Imagine how much of your on-line existence will need to be terminated. Similarly, combinations to a safe—whether an in-home safe or a storage unit with a combination lock—should be documented and retrievable. What if you had valuable personal items in an expensive safe? Avoid having loved ones call a locksmith in order to drill through the lock. Recording this information in a safe manner, and confiding its whereabouts to a trusted loved one, friend or attorney, will be extremely helpful to those who will have to sort through such details after you are gone.

In Summary

Taking the time to express messages to your loved ones, recording your needs for personal care, and writing your hopes for how your life can best be honored not only informs your decision-makers, but can also be a source of great comfort for those you love most. Consider adding these personal details to your healthcare directive.

Additionally, take a moment to consider all of the tasks that your loved ones will face after you are gone. Communicating the whereabouts of important documents, on-line access information, safe combinations, secret storage places, and the like can avert tremendous frustration. You can ease the work and the emotional strain by putting your affairs in order.

HOW

How do I make my wishes known?

Follow a process that is thorough, and includes multiple conversations.

Select a tool that meets your needs.
Ask for feedback from your healthcare provider,
healthcare agents, loved ones, and others.

Make it legal.

Execute your finished document, following the laws
in your state to have it witnessed and/or notarized.

Communicate, communicate, communicate.

Communicating your end-of-life preferences is a generous
act that ensures loved ones can honor your wishes while
loving and supporting you and each other.

Make sure your healthcare directive is accessible when it is needed.

On-line storage is highly recommended. Give access to those
you choose, or give them paper copies.
Make certain your directive is included in your medical record.

10

Writing and Communicating Your Directive

This chapter provides practical suggestions for completing the process of writing your healthcare directive. Several of the recommendations have been stated previously, but are incorporated here as part of a clearly scripted process. Take a deep breath. Walking through this process may seem overwhelming. But if you follow the recommended steps, and take your time for thoughtful consideration and for meaningful conversation, you will succeed in creating and communicating a meaningful healthcare directive.

Writing your directive once does not address your needs for all time. Reviewing and refreshing your directive every year or two will ensure your most current thinking is reflected in your healthcare instructions and that your chosen healthcare agent and your alternate agents are still available and appropriate to serve in the important role of your advocate. Refreshing your document will take significantly less time than initially creating the directive. See the suggestions under *Step 10: Keep It Current* below.

Conversation is incorporated into most steps of this process. Every conversation will contribute to successfully completing a directive that reflects your wishes, and can be honored by loved ones, healthcare professionals, and healthcare agents.

> The process of writing a meaningful directive can take days or weeks, and includes multiple conversations that may lead to revisions. Take the time to get it right.

Step 1: Choose a tool

To begin the process, you need to select a tool to use. Just like choosing the right vehicle for a family trip (small and economical or large SUV with lots of space), you need to choose the right tool to meet your needs. If you are young and healthy, a brief form may suffice. If you have a serious condition or chronic disease, select a tool with questions that are both broad and deep, in order to create a thorough healthcare directive. Remember, this is more than checking a couple of boxes. Review the forms you find and ask yourself whether all of the topics covered in this book can be addressed effectively. Various sources for healthcare directives are noted below.

> A variety of tools exist to assist you in writing your healthcare directive. Choose a tool that will allow you to communicate all of your preferences.

A. On-line tools and services. A variety of Internet-based companies offer services to help individuals create a healthcare directive. Be careful. Some simply offer yes/no/maybe answers to each question. Some do not actually comply with each state's legal requirements, but rather offer a one-size-fits-all-states approach. Some will mail you a paper form.

Some allow you to create the directive document **only** once, while others allow you to return to a website to make changes over time. As always, remember the adage, "You get what you pay for." Consider the importance of this document and its value to you and your loved ones. Then, choose carefully. Here's what to look for if you are comparing on-line options:

- Questions that address all of the topics discussed in the "What" section of this book,

- Flexibility in how you can answer questions (more than yes/no/maybe),

- The option to electronically and securely store and retrieve your healthcare directive,

- The option to easily update your directive over time,

- A healthcare directive that actually meets individual state laws instead of a one-size-fits-all approach.

> NOTE: A word of caution—some services make the statement, "We take the position that this document is legal." Be careful. Just because they take the position does not make it so. If there is a family disagreement or conflict with a physician over the treatment to provide, having a document that can be legally scrutinized and enforced is essential.

Two services are noted below:

www.PlanWellFinishWell.com. As stated earlier, my work regarding end-of-life decisions began with creating a practical approach to wrestling with these difficult decisions. Plan Well Finish Well is a website that offers tools to assist you in writing a directive.

www.agingwithdignity.org. This website offers a popular tool called "Five Wishes." A well-designed paper form is available to be completed by hand, or a fill-in PDF can be purchased. This tool is published in multiple languages and has been adopted by many hospitals around the country.

Various legal websites and medical websites offer printable forms as well. Use the Internet to search and locate other on-line options.

B. State websites. Visit your state's website and search for "advance directive" or "healthcare directive." Most states offer access to a free, no-cost form. Using a state-recommended form ensures your directive will meet the state's statutes. The disadvantage is that most state forms are very limited. Many are written with the focus on refusing treatment. Few, if any, incorporate broader topics, such as messages to your loved ones, your needs for personal care, how you define a mean-ingful quality of life, or how your life can be celebrated. Most do not address a provision for care if you develop advanced dementia. If cost is a constraint, you can certainly add an addendum to a state form to include a broader reflection of your medical and non-medical preferences, values, and beliefs.

C. Hospitals. Any hospital that receives Medicare or Medicaid reimbursement is required by law to offer a healthcare directive form to admitted patients. In some cases, the hospital includes a simple form as part of a series of forms on a clipboard handed to the patient at admission. There might even be a checkbox that states, "I do not have a healthcare directive, and I am not writing one at this time."

Thankfully, some hospitals have embraced the importance of healthcare directives and have established Advance Care Planning departments. These hospitals typically have trained facilitators on staff who will talk with you to help you identify and articulate your preferences. Often, facilitators are social workers, nurses, or in some cases, community volunteers. This can be invaluable, particularly if you are nearing the end of your life and have health conditions and complexities that require comprehensive medical advice. While a facilitator may not be able to answer a question, he or she most likely can put you in touch with a person who can address your concerns.

D. Attorneys. While a healthcare directive is a legal document, its content and format are intended to be usable by anyone, without requiring the assistance of an attorney. However, an attorney may be extremely helpful for some individuals. If you are a cautious person and like to have everything buttoned-down, having your attorney review and possibly revise your draft directive may be wise. If you have highly-charged family relationships, then it may be best to have an attorney either write your directive, or, at a minimum, review a directive you have written.

If you have adult children who may object to honoring your wishes, particularly if you have named a spouse (especially from a second marriage) as your healthcare agent, you may want to add legal language and weight to your document.

Generally speaking, attorneys in the elder law specialty are more versed in the nuances of healthcare directives than are estate-planning attorneys. Estate and trust attorneys are primarily focused on preserving wealth by navigating the complexities of tax law. Most estate attorneys describe their practice as highly technical. Thus, be careful in selecting an attorney. Find one who truly understands the value of writing a thoughtful healthcare directive, as well as one who recognizes the emotional and spiritual value of maintaining family harmony through a well-crafted directive.

E. Faith community. Many faith communities offer end-of-life preparation assistance. Resources may include conversations with a clergy-person or a trained facilitator, periodic seminars, and/or access to healthcare directive forms.

Step 2: Complete a draft

You might begin by answering the easy questions first—name, address, birth date and the like. Look over the form and understand the sections. Look at the signature pages to anticipate whether you will need witnesses or a notary public.

I recommend completing one topic or section at a time. Unless you are using a very brief form, don't try to write your entire directive in one sitting. Take your time. Set your draft aside for a few days. Come back to revisit and revise as needed. Recognize this is a draft that is subject to change.

Step 3: Talk with a trusted loved one

Once you have a solid draft, discuss your wishes with your closest loved one, most likely your spouse or partner. As you walk through the decisions, you could find instructions that need more clarification, or you might even change your mind about a decision based on your loved one's reaction. Revise your draft accordingly.

If you find it difficult to open the discussion, you might begin by simply saying "I need your help with something important." Chapter 11 offers many suggestions and techniques to help you get started. The internet can also be a source of conversational tools.

In 2010, a group of concerned media, medical, clergy, and legal professionals gathered to share their experiences regarding end-of-life conversations and decision-making. From their efforts, a grassroots, national public service campaign emerged. The Conversation Project is dedicated to helping individuals and families to talk about their end-of-life wishes for care. Kitchen table conversation is encouraged through a series of steps entitled "Get ready," "Get set," "Go," and "Keep going." This non-profit was co-founded by author and nationally recognized columnist Ellen Goodman, and Len Fishman, who served as commissioner of Health and Senior Services in the cabinet of New Jersey Governor Christine Todd Whitman and was president of the American Association of Homes and Services for the Aging.

You may make amazing discoveries as you share your ideas about end-of-life choices with your spouse or partner. Expressing your uncertainty, and bantering about the possibilities, is best done in the privacy of your closest relationship. You may learn that your spouse is unwilling to abide by one of your proposed preferences. If so, you can either make an adjustment now, or consider choosing someone else as your healthcare agent. Alternatively, you may find you are like-minded. Many couples find the conversation affirms their love and commitment, making them evermore grateful for each day they share.

John and Denise married about four years ago; a second marriage for both. Their children are all grown. John is in his mid-seventies, and has recently experienced some medical challenges. Denise, in her late fifties, is healthy.

An interesting shift occurred as John and Denise shared their healthcare directives. John expressed his desire to allow for a natural death if he should experience a significant stroke beyond his eightieth year. John cared for his father after he suffered a stroke, and watched his intelligent, vibrant father reduced to bedridden care, with little ability to communicate. John does not want to follow in his father's footsteps.

In their conversation, John asked Denise not to pursue aggressive treatment after a heart attack or stroke if he was eighty years old or beyond. She responded that if any of John's children were present and part of the discussion, she would be unable to follow his wish. Denise was unwilling to be the stepmother who allowed John to suffer pain or die in front of his children without making an effort to have medical intervention.

This revelation caused John to alter his directive to more explicitly record this instruction. He made it clear that if this scenario occurred, Denise was simply honoring his wishes. Moreover, it caused John and Denise to call a family meeting with all of their grown children to openly discuss their healthcare directives.

Step 4: Talk with your healthcare professional

Schedule an appointment with your healthcare professional (physician or nurse practitioner). Consider including your spouse or partner as a second pair of ears, so you both hear the same information from your physician. As you walk through your wishes, your doctor can affirm your choices, challenge your decisions, or supply additional facts that could cause you to make another choice. Revise your draft accordingly.

Several objectives should be addressed when you speak with your healthcare professional:

A. Be informed. Explore your options. The medical possibilities and complexities at the end of life are infinite. This book does not attempt to address individual situations. Consulting with your physician as you craft your decisions can be tremendously beneficial, particularly if you are suffering from a condition or disease or have multiple health issues. Ask questions. Share your feelings about how you define a meaningful quality of life. Your provider can elaborate on the possible outcomes for your stated preferences or might ask questions that will enable you to clarify your wishes.

Don't expect this person to discuss all of the content of your directive (messages to loved ones, personal care, celebrating your life). That's okay. Focus on the medical decisions— such as the level of intervention you would desire, the use of C.P.R., receiving artificially administered food and fluids, and your intentions for comfort care.

Your conversation may lead you to make changes to your healthcare directive document. That's great! Or, it may affirm your thinking. The more educated you are about the medical ramifications of your decisions, the more confident you can be that you are making the right choices for you.

B. Complete doctor's orders. If your circumstances warrant, discuss with your physician completing a D.N.R. and/or a P.O.L.S.T. Make certain the instructions on these forms match the instructions in your healthcare directive.

C. Find out if your healthcare provider will honor your wishes. It is critical that your healthcare provider understands and will honor your wishes. A physician can refuse to abide by a healthcare directive on the basis of:

- Personal conscience,

- Doubting the validity of the directive document,

- Professional opinion that the treatment is not medically appropriate.

In countless cases, physicians refuse to abide by an individual's directive because the physician disagrees. This is particularly common if the individual wishes to allow for a natural death, but the physician feels he might be able to save his patient, or add time to the patient's life. Hospitals receiving Medicare reimbursement (thus virtually all hospitals) will transfer a patient to another physician or hospital, at the request of the healthcare agent, if the attending physician or hospital is unwilling to adhere to the patient's healthcare directive. Researching alternative hospitals or physicians in advance of a transfer is advised to ensure the same dilemma does not recur.

Most states' statutes include a provision that allows a physician or hospital to refuse to follow a healthcare directive if they believe in good faith that the healthcare directive is not legally valid. There can be circumstances when a physician appropriately questions the legality of a directive. Sadly, forgery occurs, and sometimes family members can dupe vulnerable or elderly patients by crafting a directive that requests a natural death. However, physicians can also use this provision to ignore a legitimate request and legally documented instruction to allow a natural death.

Be proactive. Ask your healthcare provider now whether he will adhere to your wishes. Ask if he will refuse to bow to a frightened family member who requests all possible treatments if you, in fact, have written your directive to allow a natural death in certain circumstances. Equally important, ask if your physician will honor your wishes to extend your life with all possible treatment if a loved one is too quick to ask for treatments to be withheld, in spite of your directive. Physicians face tremendous pressure from well-meaning family members who may be emotionally unprepared to let you go. In the opposite scenario, less-than-honorably-motivated loved ones could pressure your physician to let you go too soon. Prepare your physician by sharing the names of individuals you worry might create conflict. Ask your physician to actually sign your directive document (a final version, after you've made any revisions).

If your physician won't agree to abide by your wishes, it is far better that you know now. Make certain your healthcare agent knows about your current physician's position. He may need to strongly serve as your advocate, even being willing to engage legal counsel to press your healthcare provider into abiding by your directive. A transfer to another physician or hospital could become necessary. Could your healthcare agent anticipate this situation? Or, would you be better served to find a new physician for your end-of-life care? If so, be sure to update your document to reflect a different physician's contact information (if included in your form).

D. Protect your healthcare provider. Most states have laws that protect a physician who is following a patient's healthcare directive. However, physicians may fear a threatened lawsuit from a family member. It is a common occurrence. Consider giving your attorney's name to your healthcare provider to elicit legal support if necessary. And, do your best to uncover any potential landmines now in a family meeting. Be proactive about helping your loved ones understand your desire to die on your terms—not theirs.

E. Share your communication expectations. Assume for the moment that you will be fully competent and able to communicate your healthcare decisions. Talk with your physician about how best to communicate with you. Do you want all the details, both positive and negative? Or do you want the rosy version? Do you give permission to talk openly about death and the dying process? Answer all of those same questions regarding communication with your loved ones. How should your healthcare provider communicate with them? Is he willing to help your loved ones recognize when you have actively entered the dying process? Will he compassionately explain the signs, helping your loved ones accept the reality of the situation?

F. Ensure your healthcare provider will be forthcoming with your healthcare agent. Research shows the majority of physicians present the optimistic view of a patient's prognosis far more readily than the negative. They are trained to solve the problem and fight the enemy of death. Acknowledging death is surrendering, and it runs against the grain of many, if not most, healthcare professionals. Thus, many providers are reluctant to share the risks and possible negative outcomes of proposed treatments. Because you are asking your healthcare agent to make decisions on your behalf, your agent needs to be fully informed. Remember that approximately 50 percent of us will need a healthcare decision made on our behalf at some point in our life. Encourage your physician to be forthright about all the positive and negative consequences of treatment choices when meeting with your healthcare agent so the best possible decision can be reached.

G. Make the investment to meet with your healthcare provider. Be advised that your appointment to meet with your physician may not be covered by insurance, including Medicare.

You may recall the political fallout of the 2008 election year. At that time, Congress was evaluating a proposal to expand Medicare to better reimburse physicians for appointments with patients to discuss end-of-life healthcare preferences. The candidates and pundits hijacked a proposal to reimburse physicians for time spent with patients discussing end-of-life wishes. Sadly, the concept of paying for advance planning was twisted into perceived sanctioning of death panels. The medical community quickly commented that this political maneuvering was an enormous disservice to our country and raised the issue: If a physician can be reimbursed for recommending chemotherapy for a terminally ill patient, shouldn't she be reimbursed for helping patients accept a terminal diagnosis and embrace comfort care and hospice, so they can experience a better quality of life in their final months, weeks, or days?

While an appointment with your provider will most likely be an out-of-pocket cost, consider this an investment to ensure your healthcare instructions are well informed and contain preferences your physician can and will honor. Who knows— the continuing debate over healthcare reform may one day lead to physician reimbursement for advance care planning, eliminating the out-of-pocket cost for patients to proactively plan for end-of-life care in partnership with their doctor or nurse practitioner.

Step 5: Elicit valuable insight

Additional conversations with your attorney and clergy-person can be helpful. While optional, they could offer valuable insight and feedback. Revise your document accordingly.

A. Attorney. If you have an estate plan, it may be appropriate to offer a copy of your healthcare directive to your attorney. As stated above, an attorney can offer suggestions for strengthening your document, particularly if your family dynamics might be challenging at the end of your life. Furthermore, your attorney can assist you in creating a Financial Power of Attorney document to ensure your financial responsibilities can be managed if you are unable to do so.

B. Clergy-person. Meeting with your clergy-person can affirm that your choices align with your faith traditions. While optional, this conversation may be the most profoundly helpful. Are you spiritually ready for the end of your life, whenever it may come? Do you have questions? Do you have a desire to explore faith matters more seriously? Additionally, this conversation can help you to elicit your clergy-person's support, both for you and for your loved ones, through the dying process. In turn, this will empower your clergy-person to engage your family in supporting your choices, should your directive be invoked in the future.

Step 6: Talk with your healthcare agent and alternates

I realize I have already expounded on the virtue of speaking to your healthcare agent, but it is so important. This recommendation is repeated as part of the process outlined in this chapter.

When I read that the *majority* of healthcare agents had no prior conversation with the patient regarding end-of-life preferences, I was startled. In fact, most agents did not even know they had been appointed to this role, much less given the opportunity to accept or decline. Summon the courage to discuss your preferences now with your chosen agent and alternates. Optimally, gather all your agents together so everyone receives the same information.

When you appoint a person as your healthcare agent or alternate, you are asking them to take on a solemn and potentially very difficult responsibility. You can ease the weight of this mantle by being forthright and sharing your intentions both verbally and in the written document. Give them each a copy and ask them to read it. Then walk through your healthcare directive in person, giving ample opportunity for each agent to ask questions. Be sure you ask questions to check each agent's understanding of your wishes. Give scenarios or examples and ask how each would respond. Clarify, clarify, and clarify some more. Revise your document, if warranted.

When you have a final version of the document, ask your healthcare agent and alternates to sign it to demonstrate their commitment to honor your wishes. Though not legally required in most states, some forms offer space for these signatures.

Step 7: Talk with your loved ones

By this point, your wishes should be clearly defined in your own mind. Discuss your wishes with your loved ones. Make additional revisions based on feedback from your circle of loved ones, as warranted. Some suggestions are noted below.

A. Have a family meeting. Not only will it ensure a shared understanding of your wishes, it will allow you to go through the process once, rather than needing to repeat it. If you show any ambivalence in front of your loved ones, it could create tremendous conflict later on, so it's best to have this conversation when you have reached a point of comfort with your own preferences, and feel you can strongly convey your wishes. For some families, this could be difficult, with possibly unpredictable results. Consider inviting a trusted friend or advisor (therapist, social worker, or clergy-person) to facilitate the family meeting with you, helping the conversation stay on track. As mentioned previously, many hospitals have advance care planning experts who may be able to facilitate the discussion. By involving everyone in the conversation, you can ensure consistency; they will all hear the same message. Be open. Be patient. But be firm with your wishes. You may wish to go so far as to ask your loved ones to sign your directive, indicating they agree to honor your wishes.

From a practical point of view, it may be difficult to host a meeting with everyone being physically present. Consider using technology to facilitate a virtual meeting. For example, a video chat session with multiple family members could be sufficient to accomplish your goal of sharing your wishes.

B. Address potential future conflict now. Perhaps one of your children, or a spouse, might be unable to withdraw treatment, if required. Therefore, you've chosen someone else as your primary healthcare agent. You can avoid hurt feelings in the future by articulating your reason for selecting someone else for your healthcare agent now. Perhaps you have children who will have great difficulty letting you go when the time comes. What if some family members espouse the sanctity of life above all else and would fight for you to receive all possible care, even against your wishes? Talk about it now. Help them understand your desire not to linger in suffering if your health should slowly decline. Equally possible, you could be a fighter. You could want every possible treatment, creating every opportunity for your recovery. Would all of your family members support your agent's pursuit of aggressive treatment? Discuss this openly.

C. Blended families, take note. Blended families are the highest source of end-of-life-related lawsuits. Though mentioned previously, it bears repeating. If you are part of a blended family, you can mitigate potential disaster by ensuring adult children understand your choices and the selection of your spouse (their step-parent) as your healthcare agent. Empower your spouse in front of your adult children. Ask for their respect, and point out the courage it may take for your spouse to abide by your wishes. Alternatively, you may find it wise to select an adult child as healthcare agent, removing this burden from your spouse. If you name both your spouse and your adult child/children, be absolutely certain you have one individual as the final authority, and explain why you've made that selection.

Step 8: Execute your directive document

When your document is finalized, including any changes made based on feedback from your physician, healthcare agents, or loved ones, the document must be executed to be made legal. Rules differ by state regarding what is required to execute a healthcare directive. Some states require two witnesses. Some states require only one witness. There are rules about who can serve as a witness. Other states require a notary public. Some states allow witnessing or a notary public. Rules are different if you live in a long-term care facility. It is confusing. If you are using your state's form, the requirements will be spelled out. You can use the Internet to search for your state's rules, or contact your attorney.

Here is a list that covers most states' restrictions on who can serve as a witness. You *cannot* choose someone:

- Already appointed as your healthcare agent,

- Directly or indirectly responsible for providing your health care. This includes your healthcare provider, an employee of your healthcare provider, or the operator or employee of a community-care facility or residential-care facility where you are receiving care,

- Related to a person who is providing your health care,

- Responsible for paying for your medical care,

- Related to you by blood, adoption, or marriage,

- Employed by your life insurance or health insurance company,

- Entitled to any part of your estate,

- Younger than eighteen years of age.

Consider having both witnesses and a notary sign your document to reinforce the deliberate nature of your effort to record your end-of-life healthcare wishes. Furthermore, this increases the likelihood that physicians from another state will honor your document should you be injured or become ill away from home.

Your healthcare directive will only be recognized as a legal document if it is properly executed. Using both a notary and two witnesses provides the greatest legal strength.

As part of executing your directive, consider eliciting optional signatures, as suggested previously in this chapter. Your healthcare agent and alternates, your healthcare provider, and your closest loved ones could all be invited to sign your directive to indicate their commitment to honor your end-of-life wishes.

Step 9: Make sure your directive can be found

Many of the recommendations listed below have already been presented in this book. They bear repeating. By definition, if your healthcare directive is needed, it is because you cannot communicate. Your directive will serve and protect you only if it can be found when it is needed. Consider the following:

A. Use secure, on-line storage for your documents; it's your best choice.

- Insist upon having 24/7 access from a computer or smart phone to ensure the most ready retrieval of your document. Furthermore, if you make changes, you can have the confidence that your most current document will be used by your agent and medical team.

- Use a state registry. Several states offer a free service where your healthcare directive can be stored through a registry available to all hospitals and physicians in your state. If you choose this option, be sure to explore what access is available if you should fall ill or be injured away from home.

- Search the Internet for other available on-line storage services.

B. Do *not* put your healthcare directive in your safety deposit box. This is a common mistake. When the document is needed, time is of the essence. On-line retrieval affords immediate access. If you prefer paper, copies should exist and be easily retrievable, as the remaining instructions indicate.

C. Update your in-case-of-emergency (I.C.E.) record in your wallet or mobile phone. Include your healthcare agent and alternates' contact information as well as your own. Also include the location of your healthcare directive, whether in paper form or as a link to a secure on-line storage site.

D. Keep a wallet card. In addition to your I.C.E. record, you may also want to keep a card in your wallet that states you have a healthcare directive and how it can be accessed. Include the name and contact information of your healthcare agent and alternates.

E. Ensure the appropriate stakeholders (healthcare agents and physician, at a minimum) can immediately retrieve your directive. "Immediately" means within five minutes. If access is electronic via the Internet, ensure those who should have access have clear instructions, including the website address and a password to access your account. If you prefer paper copies, make sure those who need copies have them. Advise your stakeholders to keep this document in a location that is quickly accessible. Keep a list of those who have a copy, in case you wish to revoke your directive in the future and need to destroy old versions.

F. Make sure your physician has your healthcare directive in your medical chart. This is a critical step to ensuring your wishes will be followed and cannot be overstated.

This may be in the form of a paper copy or as a link to the on-line storage of your directive. Take the initiative to ensure your directive is in your chart. Ask to see it reflected in your chart. Can a physician who might be under pressure easily view the details or are they buried? Is the contact information for your selected agent readily accessible? If you move to a new health-care provider, make sure your directive is included in your new medical record. If you and your physician have taken the further step of writing a D.N.R. order or a P.O.L.S.T., be sure these are also reflected in your medical record.

G. Keep a copy on your refrigerator if you are severely ill or elderly, particularly if you have a P.O.L.S.T. or D.N.R.

order. That is the first place an E.M.T. is trained to look. Purchase a plastic folder that closes, and use magnets, Velcro, or tape. Fancier versions of refrigerator-mounted folders can be found on the Internet.

H. Also keep a copy near your bed or on your bedroom door (E.M.T.s are also trained to look there) if you are severely ill or elderly. Purchase a plastic folder that closes and attach it to someplace visible on your bed or bedroom door with Velcro or tape.

I. Take copies of your documents with you when you travel. Some choose to have a copy of their directive documents in their purse or briefcase. Consider scanning the documents and keeping them on your mobile phone as a PDF in case Internet access is limited.

J. Communicate with your local E.M.T. service and local hospital if the end is near (within the next six to twelve months). For those who are severely ill or those who are very elderly, consider speaking with the E.M.T. service nearest your home and/or the hospitals most likely to care for you in a crisis. For example, while my primary physician practices at one hospital, in an emergency I would most likely be transported to a different hospital closer to my home. Having your directive on file at hospitals and E.M.T. services nearby can be tremendously helpful in a crisis. Learn whether they require a P.O.L.S.T. or Out-of-Hospital D.N.R. to honor a preference for comfort care only. Ask if both the E.M.T.s and the emergency room records can reflect "Comfort care only" in their system records, if that is your choice.

K. Share with many or just a few. Some people choose to share a copy or give on-line access to their directive to many loved ones. Other folks prefer not to involve so many people, preferring to manage the sharing of rather personal and private information. That's an individual decision. If you have taken the time to have a family meeting, additional sharing may be unnecessary.

- Make your healthcare directive easy to access quickly for those who need it. On-line storage is recommended.
- Be certain a copy is in your medical chart.
- Post your directive in a prominent location at home so emergency personnel can find it.

Step 10: Keep it current

Resolve to review your directive every couple of years. As your life brings changes, your thoughts about end-of-life treatment decisions may evolve. Additionally, several life events can cause changes in one's perspective, including: divorce, death of a loved one, decline in health, or the diagnosis of a disease or condition. Any of these events creates an opportunity to reflect upon your preferences and your selection for healthcare agent. If you make changes to your directive, provide an updated executed copy to all applicable parties. Make certain prior copies are destroyed. Better yet, use on-line storage as noted above so the most current version of your executed healthcare directive is always easily retrieved when needed.

Finally, it can be helpful to let your healthcare agent and alternates know you have reviewed your directive, and your wishes are still current. Send them an e-mail or written note to document this, with the date clearly recorded, just in case your loved ones or physician doubt whether your directive is a current reflection of your wishes.

Review your healthcare directive every couple of years, or when a major life event occurs, to ensure the document still accurately reflects your wishes.

In Summary

Yes, I have listed many steps. A checklist is available at the end of the book to make it easy to check off each step as you go. Make the necessary discussions enjoyable by planning to have special time with loved ones, taking the time to strengthen relationships. Share memories. Grow closer to those you love. Remember you are giving them the gift of peace of mind, even if the road is a bit bumpy as you deliver the gift.

Plan to complete the process through the course of weeks or even months. It is not a race. However, if you are gravely ill and time is of the essence, focus on communicating your preferences verbally, and then quickly selecting a healthcare agent.

See the opportunity, and accept the responsibility to ensure those who surround you at the end of your life are well-informed about your preferences. With a clear understanding of your intentions, your medical team and your healthcare agent will be equipped to make the best decisions on your behalf, should that be necessary. They will be able to honor your care decisions without the turmoil of family conflict and arguments. No one will threaten to sue your physician or nurse practitioner. Your loved ones will be able to love and support you through the process. Yours can be a good death.

11

Great Conversation Starters

Throughout *My Voice, My Choice,* I have encouraged you to discuss your end-of-life healthcare preferences with your healthcare provider, healthcare agents, and loved ones. Over and over, I have emphasized the value of communicating your end-of-life decisions. This chapter repeats that mantra, but does so by getting far more concrete by suggesting conversation starters.

End-of-life discussions are awkward for most of us and downright difficult for some of us. The suggestions below will help you overcome those challenges.

Proactively Planning

The best scenario is obviously to proactively plan for your healthcare directive. If you are proactively planning, you can discuss your wishes with loved ones with a lighter tone, exploring the possibilities with a slant towards a more abstract view of the document. This may make the conversation more manageable for everyone. Help those you love understand your wishes so they can honor your decisions, even during emotional turmoil.

- Be straightforward and reassure your loved ones that you are healthy. "I've asked for this meeting so I can proactively share with you my thoughts about my end-of-life healthcare preferences. I'm not sick, nor have I received any bad news. I just want to convey my wishes now while I'm healthy, when it is so much easier to discuss, rather than wait until the family is in a crisis."

- Share a story. "My friend Sally just lost her mother. When she told me the story of her mother's last days, I was so sad to hear the difficult decisions her family had to make. Sally told me the family got into a huge fight about what treatment their mom would have wanted, since her wishes weren't written down. As I listened to Sally's experience, it made me realize I've never spoken with you about my end-of-life wishes. That's why I asked you to visit today. I want to be sure my wishes are clearly known so I can spare you all unnecessary pain."

- Share your thoughts about your faith or your feelings about life after death. Let them know you want to comfort and assure them now, so they, in turn, can comfort you through the dying process. "I want you to know I am not afraid to die. I believe in life after death and see death as a natural part of life. I have written down my wishes so you will know my preferences. I know it will be a difficult time for you, but by talking about it now, I hope you'll remember this conversation, and know I am okay."

- Use this book as a springboard. Be a role model by showing how preparing for the end of life is a responsibility for each of your loved ones. "I recently read a book that taught me a lot about preparing for the end of my life. I realized I haven't communicated my preferences, and I don't know what you would want. Let's get this out in the open."

Recent Diagnosis or Medical Conditions

Perhaps you have recently received a difficult diagnosis, or maybe you have been managing your life for years with a chronic disease. In either case, you have lots of living to do. Opening up this conversation with your loved ones sooner rather than later will set the tone for honest dialogue about your choices. Families often face the greatest conflict through painful silence. In fact, there is a misplaced conspiracy of silence. Loneliness thrives in silence. Break the silence and start the conversation. Share your concerns and your fears. Invite those you love into the process of considering the end of your life. Their support could be an immeasurable blessing. Here are a few thoughts:

- Acknowledge your health challenges. "As I continue to live with [condition], I am becoming more aware of my limitations. In fact, I've been giving some thought to the end of my life. It would ease my worry if I could share my treatment preferences with you now."

- Frame the big picture. "I never would have imagined I would have been diagnosed with [condition]. It has certainly caused me to take a step back and look at my life and to consider the end of my life as well. I would like to spend some time talking about my end-of-life preferences now, as that is one way I can feel I have a sense of control."

- Make it about them. "One of my greatest concerns about living with [condition] is that I don't become a burden to you. I want to discuss my end-of-life wishes with you now, before there's a crisis, so you will know my choices. That will ease my worry about becoming a burden to you."

If the End is Near

Perhaps you are courageously reading this book, working through writing your healthcare directive because you are either rather elderly or because you have a life-limiting illness. Raising the topic of your impending passing can be exceedingly difficult. I understand. Your loved ones may be reluctant, feeling that any such discussion is insulting or a betrayal of some kind. As difficult as it is, set the tone by leading the discussion. Give your loved ones permission to lovingly and carefully explore this topic with you. Consider asking a trained advance care planning facilitator, a close friend, or even a professional such as a psychologist, clergy-person, or social worker, to guide the conversation. Here are a few thoughts:

- Let them know a conversation will ease your mind. You might begin by saying, "It would truly help me, and give me a sense of relief, if we could openly discuss my end-of-life healthcare choices."

- Share your feelings. "I feel so alone right now. It would help me to talk about the end of my life and to know you will share this time and journey with me." Or perhaps, "There is so little that I can control at this point. I would feel stronger and more in control if I knew my final wishes would be honored. Will you please listen so you will understand my preferences?"

- Consider conveying your sense of determination. "I plan on fighting this disease with all I have. Nonetheless, at some point we all will die. It is important for me to communicate my thoughts about the level of care I want to receive at the end of my life, whenever that may be."

- Frame the discussion with your concern for your loved ones. "I know how hard these past few [weeks, months] have been for you. It would help me to know that the end of my life could be less of a burden to you by letting you know now what I would prefer. I don't want you to be saddled with guessing and wondering what decisions to make if I can't speak for myself."

Bringing Up the Conversation with an Aging Parent

Here are a few thoughts for those who want to understand and honor the wishes of an aging parent. Break the silence. Take the lead. You and your parent(s) will face the dying process with greater peace and dignity for having had this conversion.

- Consider framing this discussion in a way that most honors their role as your parent. "Dad, I really need your help to get through what will be one of the most difficult times in my life when you die. I can't imagine being without you. You've always been there for me. Would you help me understand your wishes, so I can be sure I am honoring your choices? That would really ease the difficulty for me if a time ever comes when you aren't able to speak for yourself."

- Acknowledge the awkwardness and break the silence. "Mom, we've never had a chance to discuss your end-of-life healthcare choices. I don't want you to think I'm anticipating your passing. And I wonder if you've been hesitant to bring this up because you are worried it might upset me. I think it would help both of us if we could have an honest discussion instead of remaining silent."

- Address sibling differences. "Mom and Dad, it must be challenging to manage the [four] of us kids when we all see life so differently. I've started considering how the

[four] of us might view circumstances differently when each of you reaches the end of your life. If you are unable to speak for yourself, it will be so important that your treatment preferences are written down. We want to honor your wishes, instead of guessing, or even arguing with one another."

- Tell a story. "My friend Bob just went through a really difficult time with his father. Bob had to make the difficult choice to withdraw a feeding tube. He thought that's what his father would have wanted, but now he is devastated and blames himself for his father's death. I don't want to be put in that situation. I need to know what you would want if there are treatment choices to be made at the end of your life and if you can't speak for yourself."

Caring for Someone Who Is Actively Dying

Perhaps you are a caregiver or the loved one of someone who is very near the end. Allowing a dying patient to express her end-of-life wishes is an act of great generosity and grace. When both the patient and their loved ones are accepting of impending death, there can be dignity and courage in sharing the journey.

- Consider framing the discussion in a way that most honors the patient. "Your courage and dignity through this journey have inspired me. I want to honor your wishes for the end of your life, if there should be a time when you are unable to speak for yourself. I would like to really understand your preferences, and write down your wishes. Would that be alright with you?"

- Perhaps express your own emotional needs: "I am struggling with the emotions I feel, knowing you are dying. I don't want to feel any doubt or guilt about making any decisions on your behalf, if you are unable to express your own preferences. Could we please take the time together to write down your end-of-life wishes?"

In Summary

Many conversations are necessary. Storytelling can be a helpful opening. You know your loved ones. You can anticipate their responses and prepare for them. You know what works best for you. Speak from your heart. Listen with your heart. Be courageous. You will inspire others to follow your lead.

12

Getting to Yes

If you are still hesitating, you are not alone. In fact, you are joined by a majority of Americans who have not yet written a healthcare directive. Sometimes we need to stare down our objections in order to move forward. Here are several factors that can conspire to fuel our resistance, leading us to avoid any deeper thought or conversation about the end of life. Ways to respond to the concerns of a loved one, or your own objections, are offered below.

1. **Fear is the number one reason we avoid addressing end-of-life issues.** None of us can imagine suffering. By not thinking about it, we hope somehow it can be avoided. Fear is a powerful and contagious emotion.

   Developing a plan for the end of life is the best way to establish a sense of control. A plan enables us to address what we **can** control. People spend time and money to write a will to address the distribution of their stuff after they are gone. A plan to address healthcare choices while still living is even more important.

2. **Uncertainty about what comes beyond.** While spiritual faith allows many individuals to embrace life after death, others are not so sure. Uncertainty leads to discomfort, which feeds our denial.

Make peace with God. One of the greatest desires at the end of life is making peace with God or whatever you call your higher power. Why wait? Invest time in study and prayer, according to your traditions and beliefs.

3. **There's a conspiracy of silence.** Parents don't want to alarm their children by talking about death. Children don't want to offend parents by asking questions about end-of-life preferences. Spouses/partners don't want to invite conflict by raising a difficult subject.

   Be bold. Be brave. Break the silence. Be the one who establishes a new dynamic within your family to develop open and honest dialogue about the end of life. Your leadership could be a significant blessing to your loved ones in overcoming this taboo topic.

4. **We've reset our expectations for life expectancy.** Advances in medicine have extended our expected lifespan, and we've adopted the belief that most anything can be cured. Machines can keep people alive almost indefinitely.

   Define a meaningful quality of life for yourself. What does "living well" mean to you? What makes a great day? A great weekend? What would make living unbearable? Answers to these questions can help you set the boundaries for the level of medical intervention that is acceptable for you.

5. **Many of us were raised to treat doctors as if they have all the answers—and all the power.** Whatever they say goes. We'd rather leave the responsibility of the decisions

to them because we think they'll know best. This is particularly true of older generations, those presently in their seventies, eighties, and nineties.

> *Set an appointment with your doctor.* Talk about your preferences in advance. Find a doctor who will listen, who will honor your wishes, and who will work with you in partnership. Some doctors are unwilling to openly discuss end-of-life preferences. If that is your circumstance, consider finding a new doctor and working to build a trusting relationship.

6. **Many of us fear dying alone.** Remember when most families had a grandparent living with them and homes were multi-generational? Today we have far less family-centered connection with our elders than in years past. Talking about end-of-life decisions evokes the fear of loneliness.

> *Actively maintain relationships.* Talk with your family and friends about this fear. In turn, reach out to an elderly loved one or a friend who may be slipping into loneliness. Reach out to the estranged. Heal broken relationships now. "If only I had told him . . ." is such a sad realization for those grieving a loss.

7. **We are an instant-gratification, feel-good society.** It is easy to put aside wrestling through decisions that may not impact our lives for years. It's awkward and uncomfortable, so we put it off in order to deal with more immediate matters.

> *See the opportunity.* Writing a healthcare directive offers a chance to reflect on life, on relationships, and on choices to ensure a peaceful, dignified passing. It is an important investment for your future.

8. **This feels overwhelming.** We are all busy, with no time for quiet reflection about such weighty matters.

> *Accept the responsibility.* Some things in life require our attention. Writing your healthcare directive is one of them.

In Summary

Confronting objections can help you, or someone you love, move forward in writing a meaningful healthcare directive. Inaction has consequences. This is a call to courage—to overcome any objections. This is a call to action. And the time for action is now.

Conclusion:
Healthcare Directives Matter
in the Present as Well as the Future

I wish we could share a cup of coffee, relax, and get to know one another. I would love to listen through hours of conversation as you reflect upon your life and begin to consider your end-of-life wishes. As you finish reading this book, it is my sincere hope you will have a cup of coffee with those you love, sitting around the kitchen table, sharing memories and reflections.

Preparing for the end of life can be profound for some people. It affords an incredible opportunity to reflect on how your life has been, or is being, invested. For those who may be older, or those facing a recent diagnosis, it can be particularly challenging. The reality of one's mortality comes into clearer focus. For others, it is a checkmark on a to-do list. Particularly for the young and healthy, recording one's wishes may be rather abstract—a remote and distant concept. Whichever way you get there, writing your own healthcare directive is an important accomplishment.

In recent years, the language surrounding healthcare directives has shifted from a focus on the dying process to living well. Considering one's final hours, days, or weeks can serve as a catalyst to refocus and recommit to values and priorities that may have been overshadowed by the busyness of life. The first habit in Steven Covey's landmark *Seven Habits of Highly Effective People* calls us to "begin with the end in mind." That serves as a poignant and powerful reminder to reflect upon the end as part of living well in the present.

Writing your healthcare directive and reflecting upon how you will be remembered will sharpen your view of the end, which, in turn, can refocus your vision for living fully in the present.

For most people, completing a healthcare directive is as much about their loved ones as it is about themselves. Oddly enough, your healthcare directive may serve the dual purpose of enabling your loved ones to support you through the dying process, while at the same time, allowing you to support your loved ones as they struggle with your decline, and finally your death. Your instructions can ease their burden. What a powerful opportunity you have to minimize the anguish your loved ones may someday face. Moreover, your healthcare directive can lessen and even prevent family conflict.

Death can come unexpectedly. Are you ready right now? Frame end-of-life preparation with urgency. If you knew you would die tomorrow, are there:

- Relationships that need your tending now? As you consider the messages you would include to loved ones, are there people who need to hear from you now?

- People who need to know you forgive them?

- People from whom you wish to seek forgiveness?

- People you wish to thank? To express gratitude for how they have loved you, shaped you, walked alongside you?

- Emotional issues or unfinished business in your heart that needs tending?

- Life lessons and values you want to pass on in writing?

- Things you want to do to be comfortable with your own sense of spirituality? Are you at peace with God?

- Things in your worldly affairs that need to be set in order? Have you written a will, made funeral arrangements, and organized important papers so those left behind can manage the required tasks upon your death?

Preparing for the end of life affords the greatest potential for a good life as well as a good death. Several of these questions might require your attention now, as part of everyday living. Others require your attention now, as part of preparing for the end.

This message is directed specifically to Baby Boomers. We are a tsunami of future end-of-life care. We have an opportunity to redefine end-of-life care as a high-touch, personal, patient-centered experience, instead of a technology-driven, death-defying endeavor. Much like the younger generation redefined the birthing process, we can reclaim the dying process. For those who wish to receive all possible care, say so. The medical system, in its present state, works in your favor, as doctors will fight death with every tool in their arsenal. But for those who believe receiving all possible care is not compatible with a peaceful passing, for those who would choose to receive limited care or allow a natural death, make your wishes known now. While receiving the care we desire—and only the care we desire—billions and billions of dollars could be saved. By communicating our preferences to our loved ones in advance, our families can remain united while supporting us—and each other.

This book was written to raise your awareness and inspire action. Preparing for the end of your life requires self-determination. It also requires a broad perspective; *it is not just about you.* I am hopeful that you have had, or will soon have, conversations with your loved ones and your physician. The end of your life could happen tomorrow, or it could be fifty years away. Live well today, knowing you are ready for the end, whenever it may come.

Be courageous. Be prepared. Make decisions and record them in writing. Then communicate your preferences. It will give you and your loved ones peace of mind. And that's a most generous gift to all of you.

Process Checklist:
Writing and Communicating Your Directive

The following checklist is offered to help you complete the process of writing a healthcare directive. As each step is completed, check it off the list (√). For more details about each step, return to chapter 10.

1. Choose a tool

2. Complete a draft

3. Talk with a trusted loved one

4. Talk with your healthcare professional

5. Elicit valuable insight

6. Talk with your healthcare agents and alternates

7. Talk with your loved ones

8. Execute your directive document

9. Make sure your directive can be found

10. Keep it current

Step 1: Choose a tool

A variety of tools exist to assist you in writing your healthcare directive. Choose a form that will allow you to communicate all of your preferences.

Step 2: Complete a draft

Take your time in working through the questions. Complete a first draft.

Step 3: Talk with a trusted loved one

As you walk through the decisions, you could find instructions that need more clarification, or you might even change your mind about a decision based on your loved one's reaction. Revise your draft accordingly.

Step 4: Talk with your healthcare professional

Schedule an appointment with your healthcare professional (physician or nurse practitioner). Consider including your spouse or partner as a second pair of ears, so you both hear the same information from your physician. Ask questions. Communicate your preferences. Ensure your healthcare professional is willing to honor your end-of-life treatment choices.

Step 5: Elicit valuable insight

Additional conversations with your attorney and clergy-person can be helpful. While optional, they could offer valuable insight and feedback. Revise your document accordingly.

Step 6: Talk with your healthcare agent and alternates

Walk through your healthcare directive in person, optimally with all of your agents (primary and alternates) at the same time, so everyone receives the same information. Give ample opportunity for each agent to ask questions. When you have a final version of the document, ask your healthcare agent and alternates to sign it. Though not legally required in most states, some forms offer space for these signatures.

Step 7: Talk with your loved ones

Discuss your wishes with your loved ones. If necessary, make additional revisions based on feedback from your circle of loved ones. A family meeting can be extremely helpful to ensure everyone hears the same message. Use video chat technology if loved ones cannot all be physically in the same place at the same time.

Step 8: Execute your directive document

Your document must be executed to be made legal. Rules differ by state. Investigate what is required in your state. You can use the Internet to search for your state's rules, or contact your attorney. If you are using a form from your state's website, the requirements will likely be spelled out.

Step 9: Make sure your directive can be found

Your directive will serve and protect you only if it can be found when it is needed. On-line storage is recommended for the greatest level of accessibility.

Step 10: Keep it current

Resolve to review your directive every couple of years. As your life brings changes, your thoughts about end-of-life-treatment decisions may evolve. Additionally, several life events can cause changes in one's perspective, including: death of a loved one, divorce, decline in health, or the diagnosis of a disease or condition. Any of these events creates an opportunity to reflect upon your preferences and your selection for healthcare agent. If you make changes to your directive, provide all applicable parties with an updated, executed copy. Be certain to have all paper copies of the old directive destroyed.

Finally, it can be helpful to let your healthcare agent and alternates know you have reviewed your directive, and your wishes are still current. Send them an e-mail or written note to document this, with the date clearly recorded, just in case your loved ones or physician doubt whether your directive is a current reflection of your wishes.

Endnotes

1. Jane Brody, "End-of-Life Issues Need to Be Addressed," *The New York Times*, August 17, 2009 (http://www.nytimes.com/2009/08/18/health/18brod.html)

2. Ira Byock, M.D., *Dying Well: Peace and Possibilities at the End of Life*, New York, Riverhead Books, 1997

3. Monica Williams-Murphy, M.D., Kristian Murphy, *OK to Die,* MKN, LLC. 2011

4. Centers for Disease Control, "Chronic Diseases and Health Promotion" (http://www.cdc.gov/chronicdisease/overview/index.htm)

5. Betsy Murphy, FNP, CHPN, "It's About Life," *Today's Caregiver* (http://www.caregiver.com/articles/general/its_about_life.htm)

6. Madison Park, "Families Haunted by End-of-life Decisions," CNN The Chart, March 2, 2011 (http://thechart.blogs.cnn.com/2011/03/02/families-haunted-by-end-of-life-decisions/)

7. Christakis, NA, Asch, DA "Biases in How Physicians Choose to Withdraw Life Support," *Lancet*, 1993; 342, 642–646

8. Maria J. Silveira, M.D., M.P.H., Scott Y.H. Kim, M.D., Ph.D., and Kenneth M. Langa, M.D., Ph.D., "Advance Directives and Outcomes of Surrogate Decision Making before Death," *New England Journal of Medicine*, 2010; 362:1211–1218 (http://www.nejm.org/doi/full/10.1056/NEJMsa0907901#Results=&t=articleTop)

9. Alzheimer's Association. 2012 Alzheimer's disease facts and figures. *Alzheimer's and Dementia: The Journal of the Alzheimer's Association*. March 2012; 8:131–168

10. Jane Gross, "How Many of You Expect to Die?" The New Old Age, *The New York Times*, July 8, 2008 (http://newoldage.blogs.nytimes.com/2008/07/08/how-many-of-you-expect-to-die/)

11. Robert Shmerling, M.D., "CPR: Less Effective Than You Might Think," *Aetna Intelihealth*, January 3, 2010 (http://

www.intelihealth.com/IH/ihtIH/E/9273/35323/372221.
html?d=dmtHMSContent)

12. G. Brian Young, M.D., "Neurologic Prognosis after Cardiac Arrest," *New England Journal of Medicine*, 2009; 361:605–611 (http://www.nejm.org/doi/full/10.1056/NEJMcp0903466)

13. Ken Murray, M.D., "How Doctors Die," Zocalo Public Square (http://zocalopublicsquare.org/thepublicsquare/2011/11/30/how-doctors-die/read/nexus)

14. Lori Robertson, "Health Care Bill Bankruptcies," Fact-Check.org, a Project of the Annenberg Public Policy Center, December 18, 2008 (http://www.factcheck.org/2008/12/health-care-bill-bankruptcies)

15. Lisa Zamosky, "Choices at the End of Life," *Los Angeles Times*, January 22, 2010. (http://articles.latimes.com/2010/jan/22/health/la-he-end-of-life-costs25-2010jan25)

16. Betsy Murphy, FNP, CHPN, "It's About Life," *Today's Caregiver* (http://www.caregiver.com/articles/general/its_about_life.htm)

17. Angus, DC, Barnato, AE, Linde-Zwirble, WT, et al (2004) "Use of Intensive Care at the End-of-life in the United States: an Epidemiologic Study," *Crit Care Med* 32,638-643

18. Betsy Murphy, FNP, CHPN, "It's About Life," *Today's Caregiver* (http://www.caregiver.com/articles/general/its_about_life.htm)

19. Kristian Foden-Vencil, "Oregon Emphasizes Choices At Life's End," Oregon Public Broadcasting and Kaiser Health News, March 8, 2012 (http://www.kaiserhealthnews.org/stories/2012/march/08/oregon-end-of-life-care.aspx)

20. Kim Parker, "Coping with End-of-life Decisions," Pew Research Center Publications, August 20, 2009 (http://pewresearch.org/pubs/1320opinion-end-of-life-care-right-to-die-living-will)

21. Alan Meisel, "End of Life Care," *The Hastings Center*, (http://www.thehastingscenter.org/Publications/BriefingBook/Detail.aspx?id=2270)

22. Betsy Murphy, FNP, CHPN, "It's About Life," *Today's Caregiver* (http://www.caregiver.com/articles/general/its_about_life.htm)

23. Jane Gross, "How Many of You Expect to Die?" The New Old Age, *The New York Times*, July 8, 2008 (http://newoldage. blogs.nytimes.com/2008/07/08/how-many-of-you-expect-to-die)

24. "End of Life in America," *Endlink: Resource for End of Life Care Education,* Northwestern University (http://endlink.lurie. northwestern.edu/introduction/what.cfm)

25. Janet Firshein, "How Much Do We Spend on End-of-life Care?" Thirteen WNET New York Public Media (http://www.thirteen.org/bid/sb-howmuch.html)

26. Monica Williams-Murphy, M.D., Kristian Murphy, *OK to Die*, MKN, LLC. 2011

27. "Healthcare Equality Index: Advance Healthcare Directives," Human Rights Campaign (http://www.hrc.org/resources/entry/ healthcare-equality-index-advance-healthcare-directives)

28. "The Quality of Life Model," University of Toronto, Quality of Life Research Unit (http://www.utoronto.ca/qol/qol_model.htm)

29. Barry K. Baines, M.D., *Ethical Wills: Putting Your Values on Paper,* 2nd Ed., Cambridge, MA, Da Capo Press, 2006

30. State of New Jersey, Department of Health and Senior Services, "Advance Directive Forms and Frequently Asked Questions," (http://www.state.nj.us/health/advancedirective/forms_faqs.shtml)

31. "Life-Sustaining Treatment," Nolo's Plain English Law Dictionary (http://www.nolo.com/dictionary/life-sustaining-treatment-term.html)

32. Paula Span, "D.N.R. by Another Name," The New Old Age, *The New York Times*, December 6, 2010 (http://newoldage.blogs. nytimes.com/2010/12/06/d-n-r-by-another-name)

33. "Should Late-Stage Dementia Patients Receive Feeding Tubes Near the End-of-Life?" *Annals of Long-Term Care: Clinical Care and Aging.* 2011; 19(5):11 (http://www.annalsoflongtermcare.com/ article/should-late-stage-dementia-patients-receive-feeding-tubes-near-end-life)

34. Hospice and Palliative Care, "Quality of Life at the End of Life," Helpguide.org (http://www.helpguide.org/elder/hospice_care.htm)

35. Ira Byock, M.D., *The Four Things That Matter Most*, New York, Simon & Schuster, Inc., 2004

Resources

Suggested resources can be found by visiting
www.PlanWellFinishWell.com/Glossary. Resources listed
include websites, helpful books, and articles that address
healthcare directives and other end-of-life topics.

Acronyms

Here are the most frequently used acronyms in the book.
Definitions are included in the glossary below.

A.N.D.	Allow a Natural Death
C.P.R.	Cardiopulmonary Resuscitation
D.N.I.	Do Not Intubate
D.N.R.	Do Not Resuscitate
P.O.L.S.T.	Physician Orders for Life-Sustaining Treatment

Glossary

Advance care planning: a process that honors one's life, while preparing for possible healthcare decisions in the future, through a dialogue regarding end-of-life wishes. Typically, advance care planning results in the creation of a healthcare directive document.

Advance directives or an **advance directive** is a legal document that expresses the principal's end-of-life wishes. More recently, many states have adopted the term *healthcare directive* instead of advance directive. Some use *advance healthcare directive* to capture the broadest meaning of the document.

Cardiopulmonary resuscitation (C.P.R.): procedures and medications to restart and stabilize a person's heart and breathing. C.P.R. can include chest compressions, electrical stimulation to the heart, and other procedures or medication to restart the heart or maintain its rhythm. It may also include rescue or artificial breathing using intubation (ventilation) to reduce the risk of brain injury due to lack of oxygen.

Decision-making capacity: the ability to understand and make medical decisions for oneself. This is sometimes referred to as competence. Typically, this means the patient must be able to understand information about the treatment decision, use the information rationally, appreciate the consequences, and communicate a decision. The process to determine a patient's level of competence usually involves evaluation by the attending doctor, and a psychiatrist or licensed psychologist. The evaluation is usually placed in the patient's medical chart.

Do Not Intubate (D.N.I.): a written doctor's order that indicates the patient does not want to receive intubation if he stops breathing. This means the patient does not want to have a tube inserted through his airway and attached to a ventilator that mechanically breathes for him.

Do Not Resuscitate (D.N.R.): a written doctor's order that indicates the patient does not want to be resuscitated if his heart stops beating or he stops breathing. D.N.R. means the medical team should not attempt cardiopulmonary resuscitation (C.P.R.), intubation (ventilation), internal or external stimulation of the heart, or administer medications to stimulate the heart. The term D.N.A.R. is preferred by many where the "A" indicates "attempt." *Do Not Attempt Resuscitation* more accurately indicates that C.P.R. and other medical procedures are performed to attempt to resuscitate the patient and may or may not succeed.

Durable Healthcare Power of Attorney: introduced in the 1980s, this is a document in which the principal appoints the person or people who are authorized to make medical decisions on his or her behalf—if the principal is unable to make or communicate his or her own healthcare wishes. The authority given in this document is limited to healthcare decisions.

Financial Power of Attorney: a legal document in which the principal appoints a person who is authorized to make financial decisions and complete financial transactions on the principal's behalf. The authority given in this document is limited to financial matters.

Guardian: a person who has legal authority to make healthcare decisions and to manage the property *and* financial matters on behalf of another person. A guardian can be appointed by the court in the absence of a healthcare agent.

Healthcare Agent: the person(s) named by the principal in the durable healthcare power of attorney document. A healthcare agent has the legal authority to make healthcare decisions for the principal when he is unable to make or communicate his own wishes for treatment.

Healthcare Directive: a legal document that expresses the principal's healthcare wishes. It typically includes the principal's healthcare instructions and a durable healthcare power of attorney that names the principal's healthcare agent and alternate agents. Some states use the term *advance directive* or *advance healthcare directive*.

Healthcare Instructions: a document that describes treatments the principal (writer/author) wants to receive, as well as treatments the principal may want to refuse in a given situation. Healthcare instructions can include a principal's non-medical wishes and preferences at the end of life, in addition to core medical instructions.

Healthcare Proxy: a person who makes medical decisions on behalf of another person. Three types of proxies exist:

- A *healthcare agent* is the person named by the principal in the durable healthcare power of attorney document. The healthcare agent has legal authority to make healthcare decisions for the principal.
  - Sometimes this person is simply referred to as the *healthcare power of attorney,* since their authority is given in this document.
  - Some states use the phrase *healthcare representative* or *designated patient advocate.*
- A *healthcare surrogate* is a person who may be asked to make medical decisions in an emergency, when the principal has not written a healthcare power of attorney, or the healthcare agent cannot be reached. A spouse, adult child,

sibling, parent, or close friend may be asked to serve as the surrogate. This person may also be called a ***designated decision-maker.*** Medical personnel can, by default, serve as the surrogate if no one else is available.

- A ***guardian*** or ***conservator*** is a person who may be appointed by the court if an appropriate surrogate is not available. Typically, a guardian or conservator has broader powers, including the ability to manage financial decisions as well as medical decisions.

Life-sustaining Procedure: any medical procedure, treatment, or intervention that utilizes mechanical or other artificial means to sustain, restore, or supplant a spontaneous vital function. These procedures can include, but are not limited to: assisted ventilation, renal dialysis, surgical procedures, blood transfusions and the administration of drugs, antibiotics and artificial nutrition and hydration.

Living Will: a legal document intended to record the principal's wishes for types of healthcare treatment. The concept of a living will was introduced in 1969 by Luis Kutner, an Illinois attorney. Early living will forms were designed primarily to reflect the principal's desire to have treatment withheld or withdrawn if the principal faced an incurable, irreversible disease or condition. Some have broadened in scope.

Medical Power of Attorney: see Durable Healthcare Power of Attorney

M.O.L.S.T.: Medical Order for Life-Sustaining Treatment. This is a document written as a doctor's orders for end-of-life treatment.

> Note: Various states and/or hospitals also use the acronyms M.O.S.T., P.O.L.S.T. and P.O.S.T.

M.O.S.T.: Medical Order for Scope of Treatment. This is a document written as a doctor's orders for end-of-life treatment.

Patient Self-Determination Act: legislation passed by Congress in 1990. This act gives patients the right to facilitate their own healthcare decisions, and to accept or refuse medical treatment of any kind. It requires healthcare delivery systems (hospitals, nursing homes, hospice providers) to:

- Ask each admitted patient if they have a healthcare directive.
- Include a copy of the directive in the patient's chart, if a copy is provided by the patient.
- Offer information about healthcare directives, including information about the patient's right to refuse treatment.
- Make a healthcare directive form available.
- Explain the hospital's policy on following a patient's healthcare directive.
- Facilitate the transfer of a patient to another physician or hospital if the attending physician or hospital is unwilling to adhere to the patient's healthcare directive.

P.O.L.S.T.: Physician Orders for Life-Sustaining Treatment. This is a document written as a doctor's orders for end-of-life treatment.

P.O.S.T.: Physician Orders for Scope of Treatment. This is a document written as a doctor's orders for end-of-life treatment.

Principal: the author/writer of a healthcare directive.

About the Author

Professionally, **Anne Denny** has served as a consultant in the healthcare industry for sixteen years. Her personal life has been deeply touched by Alzheimer's disease. Anne's mother died in May 2012 after living with Alzheimer's for twenty years. Her family experienced a long, slow journey as her mother retreated into a physical shell. The convergence of her professional expertise, the impact of her mother's journey, and Anne's heartfelt desire to contribute in some small way to society, led to the writing of this book.

Using her professional expertise, Anne began by building a web-based tool to offer a more approachable, more meaningful process for exploring and communicating our end-of-life healthcare preferences with our loved ones. She expanded her vision to reach more people by writing this book, and sharing the importance of healthcare directives through her speaking engagements.

Anne brings both her professional and her life experience to *My Voice, My Choice*. Anne's passion is clear: "I have a heartfelt desire to ease the burden of end-of-life decisions for loved ones, as well as helping individuals to approach the end of life with less uncertainty and fear."